Successful Ageing

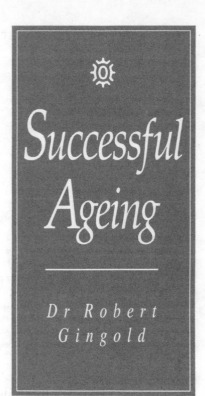

Successful Ageing

Dr Robert
Gingold

Melbourne
OXFORD UNIVERSITY PRESS
Oxford   Auckland   New York

OXFORD UNIVERSITY PRESS AUSTRALIA

Oxford New York Toronto
Delhi Bombay Calcutta Madras Karachi
Kuala Lumpur Singapore Hong Kong Tokyo
Nairobi Dar es Salaam Cape Town
Melbourne Auckland

and associated companies in
Berlin Ibadan

OXFORD is a trade mark of Oxford University Press

National Library of Australia
Cataloguing-in-Publication data:

Gingold, Robert, 1949–
  Successful ageing.

  Bibliography.
  Includes index.
  ISBN 0 19 553206 6.

  1. Aged — Life skills guides. 2. Ageing. 3. Old age.
  I. Title.

646.79

Designed by Sandra Nobes
Typeset by Syarikat Seng Teik Sdn. Bhd., Malaysia.
Printed in Hong Kong
Published by Oxford University Press,
253 Normanby Road, South Melbourne, Australia

CONTENTS

ACKNOWLEDGEMENTS

I wish to express my appreciation to a number of people who have helped and encouraged me during the writing of this book. Bronia Rennison for her tireless support during the researching of information. Special thanks to Dr Hal Kendig whose expertise in this topic was reflected in his invaluable and constructive comments.

The '12345+ Nutrition Plan' is the result of the research by Dr Katrine Baghurst and Ms Sally Record (CSIRO Division of Human Nutrition, Adelaide) and Professor Ann Hertzler (Virginia State University). I thank them for giving permission to include their nutritional recommendations. Dr Terry Seedsman's suggestions on exercise in later life were most helpful. I am also grateful to the following experts who patiently read and commented on the relevant parts of the text: Dr Peter Cowan, Mrs Deidre Jones, Ms Antigone Kouris, Dr Harry Lipp, Dr Robin Marks, Dr Jim Penny and Dr Roger Warne.

During my 15 years in general practice I have admired many energetic older people who live and enjoy life to its fullest. They inspired me to write this book and have taught me a lot about the art of successful ageing.

I gratefully acknowledge their contribution. I am grateful to the following people for allowing me to reproduce illustrations and/or copyright material:

Figure 2.1: Wadsworth Publishing Company, Belmont, CA 94002. *Figure 2.2:* The Early Planning for Retirement Association. *Figure 3.3:* J. Williams and M. Jelinek, 'Walking for Fitness', *Patient Management* Jan. 1990, p. 49. *Figure 4.1:* R. English, 'Towards Better Nutrition for Australians,' *Report of the Nutritional Taskforce of the Better Health Commission*, AGPS, Canberra 1987, p. 39. *Figure 4.2:* The 12345+ Nutrition Plan is the result of research by Dr Katrina Baghurst, Prof. Ann Hertzler and Ms Sally Record,

CSIRO Division of Human Nutrition, Adelaide. *Figure 5.2:*
What's Age Got To Do With It? Department of Sport Recreation and Tourism, 1987. *Figure 6.1: Statistics on Drug Abuse*
in Australia, AGPS, Canberra 1990, p. 37. *Figure 6.2:*
Reproduced with the permission of the Department of
Veteran's Affairs, Pharmacy Brancy. *Figure 6.3:* Reproduced
with the permission of Dosett®. *Figure 7.1:* G. Maddox, *The*
Encyclopaedia of Aging, Springer Publishing Company Inc.
New York 1987, p. 185. *Figure 7.2:* adapted from the brochure
Breast self-examination, Anti-Cancer Council of Victoria.
Figure 7.3: The Australian Nutrition Foundation. *Appendix*
1: D. Fonda and C. Wellings, *Urinary Incontinence — A*
Practical Guide for People with Bladder Problems, Their Carers
and Healthcare Professionals; ABCD Publishing, Melbourne
1987.

To Mary, Michael and Naomi

1 THE AGEING REVOLUTION

'Grow old with me!
The best is yet to be'
Robert Browning,
from *Rabbi Ben Ezra*

INTRODUCTION

To age successfully is the ultimate challenge. A number of physical, emotional and social changes are crowded into this time of life and these can be overcome so that later life is enjoyable and fulfilling. Throughout history there have been many examples of people who continued to make outstanding contributions in the latter part of their lives. At seventy-one Michelangelo was appointed supervising architect of St Peter's Church and started construction of its dome, still the largest in the world. Guiseppi Verdi composed *Otello* at age seventy-three, and the Australian dancer Sir Robert Helpmann, at age seventy-seven, danced Red King in *Checkmate*, a role he created forty-nine years earlier. Bertrand Russell and Bernard Shaw, both Nobel prize winners for literature, continued to write well into their eighties. Public office is also testimony to the capabilities of older people. Winston Churchill was sixty-six when he was elected Prime Minister of Britain during World War II, and Sir Mark Oliphant's five-year term as Governor of South Australia began when he was seventy.

The elderly today will live almost twenty years more than their ancestors at the turn of the century. This is a revolutionary change and is reason for celebration. The dual purpose of this book is to build on the improvements which increased our lifespans, and to encourage success in all aspects of later life. There is no room for complacency in believing that all the answers are known or that it is too late to try. Indeed, this book offers new insights and presents exciting and challenging opportunities for older people. It is intended to be not only a 'good read' but also to make a difference to the way ageing is perceived.

Ageing is a normal biological process that begins at birth. There is a great diversity in the rate people age, and chronological or calendar age can be a poor indicator. Today, despite the fact that people live longer and are healthier, social convention continues to impose retirement at sixty-five. Psychological attitudes can make the elderly feel useless at this age, although they are well and productive. Such outdated values must be replaced with the present day reality of later life.

A person functions as a whole, therefore a broad view must be taken when examining the factors that affect ageing. Diet, exercise, smoking and other lifestyle factors are important to good health. Each is discussed in detail in Chapters 3–6. In addition, occupation, housing, social opportunities, finance and friendships affect the way we age, although these are less obvious influences. All these factors are important when considering total health and the quality of later life.

The benefits of successful ageing are considerable. Improved health and fitness significantly influence a person's independence. Good health implies more than merely the absence of disease and physical wellbeing: it includes mental soundness and social satisfaction. Many illnesses are influenced by what people do for themselves, and a suitable choice of lifestyle can prevent a number of diseases from developing. Implementing these preventive lifestyle practices is the ideal way to maintain good health.

Less tangible benefits of successful ageing include a general feeling of wellbeing and a satisfaction with life. People who enjoy life are proud of their age and have high self-esteem. The desire to remain an involved and contributing member of society can be a self-fulfilling prophecy, and later life can herald all kinds of new beginnings.

VITAL STATISTICS

The importance and influence of people over sixty years of age will increase with the predicted growth of the population in future years. This has already started to occur, but will become more obvious as the post-war baby boom generation reaches old age early in the twenty-first century. These people are likely to have a profound effect on the attitudes to old age, in the same way they affected attitudes to youth during the 1960s. The ageing of the population is indicated in the following table, which gives the number of people over sixty from early this century, and the projected increase into the next century.

TABLE 1.1 The number of people over sixty from 1901

Year	Number of people over sixty (million)	%
1901	0.15	4
1947	0.6	8
1981	2	14
1990	2.6	15.4
2001	3	16
2021	5	22

The life expectancy of men and women will continue to increase, as the following figures indicate:

TABLE 1.2 Life expectancy of men and women

Year	Men	Women
1901	55.2	58.3
1989	73.3	79.5
2020	79	87

Between 1981 and 2001 the number of older people will have increased by 50 per cent, with an even greater increase in those aged over seventy. In the year 2020 men can expect to live to seventy-nine, and women to eighty-seven. They will reach later life in better health than previous generations, and the majority will live independently. The maintenance of good health into these later years will enable most to remain vital, active and robust individuals.

MYTHS OF AGEING

Youth is promoted as the best time of life — carefree and fun filled. By contrast, later life is described as the decline from a youthful peak. The reality is that at all ages there are both advantages and problems. The exuberant energy of youth is tempered by the turbulent search for one's identity, while the serenity and fulfilment of later life can be rudely interrupted by illness and grief. This chapter examines and questions widely accepted beliefs about how people live the last twenty to thirty years of their lives.

The term 'ageism' is used to describe discrimination against the aged, in the same way racism refers to racial prejudice. Words such as 'inactive', 'lonely', 'demented' and 'senile' are commonly used to describe older people. This portrays a negative stereotype which is not borne out when the facts are examined. The majority of older people live active and productive lives, remaining alert and independent individuals.

My children were surprised when I told them that I intended to go trekking in Nepal. I feel fit and have been walking regularly to train for it. I am the same adventurous person I have always been. I don't feel old and my age won't stop me from living.

Val (62)

Some of the responsibility for promoting and perpetuating these myths rests with the elderly themselves who can too readily accept this inferior and inglorious role. An attitude that in later life a person will be lonely, unproductive and helpless may result in just that. On the other hand, if a person's self-image is positive and he or she works hard towards achieving goals in areas as diverse as further education, exercise or personal relationships, then later life will undoubtedly be more enjoyable and fulfilling.

The change to a more positive attitude begins with the individual. For example, in the future it would be pleasing to see elderly people exercising in public, a sight which is rare at the present time. These individual changes multiplied many times will eventually result in a more positive attitude towards later life throughout the community. The women's movement provides a model here. The huge effort on the part of women has dramatically improved (and continues to improve) the lot of this disadvantaged group. A useful first step is to look more closely at some of the false myths relating to older people.

Ageing and Disease

One common myth is that ageing and disease are synonymous. Ageing is a normal part of the life cycle, and not a disease that is 'caught' or can be 'cured'. There are, however, many illnesses such as arthritis, heart disease and cancer that occur more frequently with advancing years, but these are entirely separate from the ageing process which alone does not result in ill health.

The idea that there is a fountain of youth, or the more 'modern' expectation of a tablet or medication to halt ageing, reinforces the myth that ageing is abnormal and must be treated. Denial of the natural life cycle serves only to limit enjoyment of the many positive aspects of later life.

A related misconception is that later life is a time of illness and incapacity. Again this stereotype is false, with research confirming that most elderly people lead independent, healthy lives. Unfortunately people frequently do accept that ill health is normal in later life, and ignore the warning signs of illness by dismissing them as part of ageing. This only delays diagnosis until the time when a problem becomes advanced and more difficult to treat. Incontinence, breathlessness and poor memory are often attributed to ageing; this is incorrect and each of these complaints warrants proper assessment and treatment. Symptoms that develop in later life are due to illness, not to age.

It is not normal to feel ill in later life. The elderly are in fact survivors who have suffered less disease than their contemporaries who have not lived to old age.

Feeble-mindedness and Dementia

Even if the body does not show changes associated with ageing it is often assumed that an older person's mental faculties rapidly deteriorate. Terms such as 'demented' and 'senile', and sayings like 'no fool like an old fool' are often used to describe an older person's intellectual capacity. This generalization is false. Even when people over eighty years of age are examined, more than 80 per cent have normal intellectual function. Of the remaining twenty per cent the majority suffer from Alzheimer's disease, which is a specific illness in the same way that heart failure is a disease of the heart. Alzheimer's disease is not normal ageing of the brain.

Forgetfulness is very common in the elderly and is due to the natural decrease in brain cells which starts about age forty. This is separate from, and does not progress to dementia. It is a benign common inconvenience and does not herald the onset of a failure in intellect and brain function.

The saying, 'you can't teach an old dog new tricks', underlines the common assumption that with age comes the inability to be educated in new areas and understand new ideas. This is another inaccurate stereotype. Many people in retirement develop new skills and hobbies which they were unable to pursue in earlier years due to the constraints of work. The University of the Third Age is a learning institution established solely for the further education of older people. Some of the greatest scholars this century, such as Bertrand Russell and Albert Einstein, continued to produce great work, their opinions sought and respected, when they were in their eightieth and ninetieth decades of life.

All the Elderly are the Same

Stereotypes reflect our tendency to group people together as an 'homogeneous mass'. In regards to the elderly, this has produced the assumption that they feel, behave and react in the same way. This is incorrect. More than at any time in the life cycle there exist significant differences and wide individual variation. At a given age (for example seventy) one person may be the president of a nation while her or his contemporary might live as a dependent invalid in a nursing home.

This massing together tends to reduce the general standard of expectation in the older age group to a lower level than they normally function at. There is a myth that most elderly people are in nursing homes or other institutional care, while in fact over 90 per cent live independently in the community. Low expectations are likely to result in low achievement, but by rejecting these stereotypes individuals are able to reach their full potential.

The Aged are Sexless

Recent research has revealed that many elderly people continue to enjoy an active sex life. It is widely believed that the elderly not only lack the desire for sex, but that they are physically incapable. Both these assumptions are incorrect. A more objective assessment reveals that it is often the children, relatives and friends dealing with the elderly who have a problem accepting and coping with the sexuality of older people. This is especially true in children where Oedipal feelings may block recognition of their parents' sexual interests. Many couples maintain an active sex life well into their seventies and eighties.

Allied to sexual feelings is the need for closeness, love and affection. These are often denied to the elderly whose physical environment and bodily functions are catered for but who are left emotionally isolated. It is important to maintain close physical and emotional contact such as being hugged and kissed. People require friendship and love, with sexuality as an integral part of an intimate relationship at all ages.

The Aged are Useless and Powerless

Present western society places emphasis on work, wealth and power. It is therefore not surprising that along with the changes that occur in later life comes the feeling that life has lost its purpose. After retirement people who were previously leaders at work and in the community perceive themselves as relegated to the 'scrap heap'. This is not true of other cultures. Tribal groups respect the wisdom of their elders, who become the powerful leaders of the community while the younger members continue with the mundane work of everyday existence. It is to be hoped that in the future changes in attitude will enable the true worth of the older members in so-called 'developed' societies to be recognized and valued.

The wisdom of life experience cannot be gained from education. The older population has a wealth of such experience which affords a lifetime perspective to current problems. In addition, they are more likely to have time to offer these services. Sadly, older people are seldom consulted by younger family members and by society in general.

What all this means, by extension, is that older people lack influence in the community. As the number of older people increases, however, their power will correspondingly grow, especially political power. More attention will then be paid and more resources allocated to this section of the community. Already groups such as the 'Grey Panthers' in the United States and 'Grey Power' in Australia are transforming political approaches to the care, health and facilities available to people in later life.

Basic Human Needs

The needs of those in later life are no less than they were in younger years. Good health, an adequate standard of living and a sense of purpose are all essential for a satisfying life at any age. Unfortunately many factors work against this. Retirement is enforced, with many people stopping work for no other reason than they have reached the magical age of sixty-five. In addition, the income from the pension is often less than a working wage resulting in a lower standard of living in later life. The elderly are entitled to equality.

UNDERSTANDING AGEING

The basic building block of the body is a single cell. Some cells have specialized functions and when grouped together form the different organs in the body. A natural turnover occurs, with old cells dying and being replaced by new ones. In childhood more cells are produced than die, resulting in growth. In the late teens and twenties there is a balance between production and loss. After thirty years the balance tips the other way, with more cells dying than can be replaced. This is mirrored in the changes in weight observed at different ages. There is rapid growth and weight gain during childhood until a balance is reached at maturity. This is followed by a gradual loss of cells and the resultant weight loss with advancing age. This process of gradual cell loss over many years results in ageing. An unhealthy lifestyle accelerates the loss of cells and hastens the ageing process. Lack of exercise, for example, results in fewer muscle cells being produced simply because they are not needed.

In the natural ageing process all the cells are normal. This differs from disease, in which some cells are abnormal. For example cancer cells look and behave differently to healthy 'old' cells. Certain drugs such as tobacco and alcohol also cause cellular damage not seen in ageing. There is therefore a clear distinction between normal 'healthy' ageing, often called 'successful ageing', and illness which is often mistaken to be part of ageing.

RESEARCH INTO AGEING

There is no proven theory to explain ageing but much research is under way to uncover the mystery. It has been suggested that humans have a maximum life span of 120 years, and it seems unlikely that life can be extended beyond this age. As we have seen, improved living standards and medical care mean that more people are living longer.

One particularly interesting observation is that different body cells have varying lifespans or ages. The red blood cells automatically die and are replaced after 120 days while brain cells age slowly over decades. When skin cells are taken from the body and grown artificially they will divide fifty times before dying. This suggests that there is some code or information in each cell that determines how long it will live.

Five of the more recent and accepted theories of ageing are discussed below.

Wear and Tear

This older idea likens the body to a machine. The 'parts' simply wear out with use, while at the same time waste products accumulate — much like rust in an old engine. Support for this theory is found in old human brain cells that contain a toxic brown pigment called lipofuscin, which may interfere with the normal function of the cell and eventually cause its death.

According to this theory, the body, like a well-maintained machine, will perform better and last longer when cared for correctly. The choice of healthy foods (fuel), avoiding alcohol and tobacco (impure pollutants), and a regular medical check-up (servicing), are all likely to result in a more healthy and robust individual (engine).

Breakdown of the Immune System

The function of the immune system is to protect the body from foreign invaders such as viruses and bacteria. It also has a role in surveillance and destruction of any abnormal or cancer cells that may arise. A poorly functioning immune system results in an increased number of infections and cancers.

Further problems arise when immune cells cannot differentiate between friend (its own body) and foe (outside invaders). This results in attacks on normal body tissues, which is referred to as autoimmunity. A number of diseases, for example rheumatoid arthritis, are due to these autoimmune problems.

The immune theory suggests that ageing is the result of a breakdown in immunity. Supporters of this theory point out that the thymus gland, which is crucial to the correct functioning of the immune system, is one of the first organs to age.

Programmed Ageing

Proponents of this theory suggest that the body has an in-built clock, or tape of information. As the tape is played a person progresses from childhood, through adolescence and on to old age. This idea certainly has some appeal, and may explain the fixed lifespan of certain cells. This is further evidenced by studies on children with progeria. This is a rare genetic disorder in which it appears the tape has been played much too rapidly. These children exhibit many of the changes and diseases found in old age including baldness, wrinkled skin and atherosclerosis (hardening of the arteries).

Central to this theory is that both beneficial and harmful characteristics are inherited, and that these characteristics determine a person's health and lifespan.

The Error Theory of Ageing

Each cell has a nucleus which contains all the information required for the normal functioning of that cell. The nucleus is comprised of strands of DNA which hold precise genetic instructions. There are a number of chemical steps involved in the process of reading the information code on the DNA and producing what the cell needs to continue living. The error theory of ageing suggests that errors in information and copying result in the production of incorrect cell requirements which interfere with normal cell functions. As a result ageing and finally death of that cell occurs. The chances of these errors spontaneously arising are more likely in older cells, as problems can occur each time reading of the DNA is performed.

A variation of this theory suggests that abnormal or damaged DNA is unable to be repaired, and that reparation is essential for the maintenance of the correct code in the cell which in turn ensures its survival. Failure to repair damage will result in abnormal DNA or mutations. Again, this wrong information ultimately causes the cell to age and die. There is a close relationship between ageing and DNA repair, with older cells less able to repair any damage.

It can be concluded then, that abnormal DNA or incorrect reading of the DNA leads to ageing. It has been known for a long time that DNA can be damaged by certain environmental factors such as chemicals and radiation. The rapid ageing of skin that has been excessively exposed to the sun is one of the most obvious effects of radiation. A simple precaution to prevent premature ageing of the skin is to protect it from the harmful rays of the sun.

The Free Radical Theory of Ageing

Free radicals also damage DNA. This accelerates ageing and leads to diseases such as cancer. These highly active free radicals are toxic forms of oxygen and are produced by the body in chemical reactions that use oxygen (oxidation). Antioxidants defend the body against these free radicals. Vitamin C, vitamin E, and beta carotene, a form of vitamin A, are naturally occurring dietary antioxidants. Experiments show that animals fed vitamins C, E and beta carotene are less likely to develop some forms of cancer.

Many antioxidants are sold commercially as anti-ageing cures. However, there is no evidence to support taking vitamins in the high doses suggested. In fact excessive intake may be harmful. High doses of vitamin E, for example, can cause diarrhoea and skin rashes. A more sensible approach is to include foods such as fruit and vegetables, that contain adequate amounts of vitamins C, E and beta carotene, as part of a balanced diet.

Experimentation on rats has also provided some interesting insights into the effects of diet on ageing. By reducing the dietary, but not the nutritional intake of food by 60 per cent, the lives of 'starved' rats were increased by 50 per cent. Although this research is important, the present level of knowledge does not lead to the conclusion that starvation be recommended as a means of prolonging life in humans. It does however raise the significant point of a possible relationship between ageing and diet. A later chapter is devoted to healthy eating.

These observations strongly suggest that disease and ageing can be influenced and possibly prevented by certain lifestyle practices, in this case a balanced diet. It supports the recommendation that a diet containing adequate vitamins and minerals, but not high in calories, is likely to result in successful ageing.

SUCCESSFUL AGEING — THE ELDERLY ELITE

There is a wide variation in the health, outlook and abilities of older people, as discussed earlier under the heading 'Myths of Ageing'. Robust individuals who remain healthy, alert and independent are described as having aged successfully. Not only do they tend to live longer but the quality of their lives is also usually superior. The question thus arises, what characteristics and attitudes do these people possess that give them an advantage over their less successful contemporaries?

The favourable attributes discussed are simply observed characteristics, often without known scientific basis. The will to live cannot be measured, but without a reason or desire for living ill health often intervenes. For instance, research shows that following the death of a spouse there is an increased incidence of illness in the surviving partner. During this grieving period feelings of loneliness and despair are common. Some feel that life alone no longer has meaning or purpose and this may lead to losing the will to live altogether. These strong emotional and social factors influence health, possibly by affecting the immune system. The exact mechanism, however, remains unknown.

There are many intangible factors that can interrupt the maintenance of good health. Science and medicine have concentrated on the physical aspects of lifestyle, encouraging people to eat healthy foods, to exercise regularly and not to smoke. While these things are important, they do not provide the total answer. We will turn now to investigate in more detail the profound effects emotions and the social environment may have on a person's health and wellbeing in later life.

The following attributes have been observed in the 'elite elderly' — those who lead active, independent and long lives.

Heredity Factors

If parents lived long healthy lives it is likely their children have inherited some of their positive genetic characteristics and will age in a similar manner. Those whose parents died at a young age (younger than sixty years) should not despair, but carefully examine all the risk factors associated with the disease that contributed to a premature death. For example, if a parent died from lung cancer which has now been conclusively linked to smoking, their children would obviously be well advised not to smoke. In such a case there is a greater chance of the non-smoking 'child' living longer than his or her parents. A healthy lifestyle then, can prevent the development of some diseases suffered in previous generations.

Being born female is another genetic characteristic that carries with it the advantage of living on average five years longer than a male. The reasons for this are unclear, with hormonal, social and psychological differences perhaps all having a role. The ideal is to be born a female, to parents who lived independently to a healthy ripe old age!

Social and Economic Factors

Financial security and education are other factors that affect ageing and longevity. People in the higher socio-economic groups generally enjoy better health. This is due to an improved lifestyle, with the ability to purchase better quality food and having the means for recreational and sporting activities. The better educated are more informed about healthy lifestyle practices and consequently suffer from less heart disease than less fortunate members of the community. Secure financial status also allows greater access to medical services. Many studies have shown that those with less income tend to smoke, eat poorer quality food, take more medication and have a higher incidence of illness. In order to improve the health and lifespan of the whole population, substantial social and economic changes over all sections of society will be needed. These changes are not reliant on further research and knowledge, but can be brought about by implementing more effectively what is already known. All people in the community, irrespective of their age or social and economic status, are entitled to good health.

Social Activities and Relationships

An active social life, whether it is involvement in family, community or work activities promotes successful ageing, and this is especially true when this is combined with a loving and caring relationship. Maintaining social contacts through family, friends, social clubs or work prevents boredom and preoccupation with one's own problems. Social isolation is a major cause of depressive mental illness in later life. To prevent this occurring it is essential to remain flexible and able to redirect activities in response to work and recreation changes as they evolve in later life. Too often retirement is simply a time of ceasing to work, leaving a void in the person's life. A more fruitful approach would be to develop interests, hobbies, voluntary or part-time work to replace the time previously spent in full-time employment.

Marriage provides emotional support and companionship. The familiarity of marriage provides stability in a rapidly changing world. In addition a spouse is a source of comfort and can provide care in times of need. It is not surprising that couples in a supportive and caring relationship tend to age more successfully. Interestingly there is often a close correlation between the lifespans of a husband and wife which may reflect their similar lifestyles.

Emotional Attitudes

A more difficult area to define is a person's mental attitude to life. Those with a positive attitude, who live independently and are able to make their own decisions on which direction their life will take, tend to be healthier people at any age. If the stereotypes of ageing are rejected and people consider themselves special and unique individuals, it is likely they will age in a distinctive and non-conformist manner.

People who retain control over their lives and make independent decisions, have less depression and fewer emotional conflicts. There is a tendency, often by well-meaning friends and relatives, to organize the lives of the elderly. This robs the older person of her or his independence and self-reliance, and results in a loss of confidence. Accommodation is a common source of disagreement. A family may decide that an elderly relative should leave his or her own home to live in what the relatives consider more appropriate accommodation. Conflict can be avoided if the older person is consulted and involved in making any major decisions of this kind.

Love is another essential ingredient for a rich and fulfilling life. The ability to love and accept oneself, 'wrinkles and all', provides a solid foundation for emotional stability. The sharing of love, both the giving and receiving, enriches interpersonal relationships. An older person must be allowed to show affection and to remain a useful member of the family. Such relationships are mutually beneficial, with the older person providing practical support for friends and family. The help may be as simple as looking after grandchildren, or more demanding, such as providing assistance in times of crisis. Such involvement gives a sense of belonging and the feeling that life has a purpose.

Many doctors and scientists believe there is a close relationship between emotional stress and the development of diseases. Stress is known to cause the release of certain hormones and influence the function of the immune system. Both of these changes are possible explanations for the link between emotional stress and physical ill health. Restating this another way is to suggest that stress and negative emotions predispose a person to disease and may even cause early death. If this is true it is not illogical to say that positive emotions — love, laughter and contentment — may prevent the development of disease and prolong life. Although the influence of positive emotions on health, wellbeing and longevity have not been extensively studied, many of the elderly who have aged successfully exhibit a positive zest for life.

Healthy Lifestyle

The diseases that are common in a community vary according to the lifestyle adopted by its inhabitants. In the developing world infectious diseases remain prevalent, while in affluent western countries like Australia, heart disease, stroke and cancer are the main causes of death. Although these diseases are individually different, the people who suffer from them frequently have in common a number of lifestyle habits. Much of the advice for preventing these diseases overlaps and most of them can be avoided by instituting similar healthy habits. These include eating a balanced diet, engaging in regular exercise, and not smoking. There is no doubt that good health enhances the quality of one's life.

2 EMOTIONAL CHALLENGES

'To be respected is the crowning glory of old age.'

Cicero

INTRODUCTION

It is remarkable to reflect on the changes that have occurred in the last half century. Society has moved from the 'horse and buggy' era to the present time when cars, computers and world-wide communication are an accepted part of everyday life. In the span of one lifetime moral values and beliefs have changed many times, with previously taboo subjects, ranging from death to homosexuality, now commonly discussed. The task of adapting to a changing world is not new to those in later life who have witnessed these dramatic changes and generally adjusted to them. If the same optimism, vigour and determination is applied to the challenges of later life, these too will be successfully overcome.

There is a widely held belief that the elderly are rigid, inflexible and incapable of change, implying that it is difficult to adapt to the challenges of ageing. We have discussed this earlier under 'Myths of Ageing', and this assumption was shown to be incorrect. There are always those who will have difficulty adapting to change, but it is probable that for these people this has been the case throughout their lives. These people are also more likely to blame 'age' for their problems in later life, thus shifting the burden of responsibility.

Every stage of life presents rewarding challenges as well as difficult adjustments. Adolescence, marriage, mid-life crisis and retirement are all important events which are often stress-ful. Much has been written on adolescence and more recently mid-life crisis, but the transition to later life has been largely ignored. Retirement, housing, grandparenthood and death of a spouse are all issues that signify it is a period of readjust-ment. Many of these changes are inevitable, and success or failure in overcoming them is often based on one's psychologi-cal reaction. The wisdom of experience, as well as learning new skills and applying innovative solutions, may be required to ensure such transitions are smooth.

Preparing for the problems that lie ahead enables people to deal with them in a more positive way. Unfortunately many people wait for circumstances to overtake them before trying to adjust to a new situation. One spouse may have taken care of all the financial affairs, for example, and on her or his death the partner may be left struggling with these matters. If such problems are anticipated, situations like this need not arise. This chapter will deal with many of the physical and emotional challenges encountered in later life.

EMOTIONAL HEALTH

The relationship between stress and ill health is generally ac-cepted. It is therefore not illogical to suggest that emotional tranquillity can influence the same process in a positive way, preventing disease and promoting a healthy long life. The points below suggest a lifestyle or approach to ageing that will help achieve these goals. While reading them keep in mind that everyone has the ability to change and incorporate these factors into their lives.

Independence

Physical independence, in not being excessively reliant on others in day-to-day living, and emotional autonomy, that enables people to make their own decisions, are equally impor-tant. While some help may be needed, it should be the support a person has decided is required, and not what others have forced upon him or her. Well-meaning family and friends often try to make important decisions in what they believe is another person's best interest, but fail to ask that person's opinion. This is particularly common in the choice of accommodation, where institutional care is often the only alternative considered. There are now many opportunities to obtain support that allow and encourage the maintenance of independence in later life. For emotional good health it is important that older people have the freedom of self-determination and retain control over the direction of their lives.

Involvement and Goal Setting

Each of us has particular strengths and talents. These may have been gained from a previous career or be new areas that have not been explored due to the constraints of work and family responsibilities. Maintaining an interest and involvement in some form of activity not only allows time to be spent more constructively but also carries with it a feeling of being useful and wanted. The scope of activities now available is enormous, ranging from all kinds of hobbies and studies, through to caring for grandchildren or starting a new job or business. Setting goals is likely to encourage people in their new endeavours. A task successfully completed brings a sense of achievement and accomplishment. This in turn is likely to build confidence, and encourage a person to greater things.

Flexibility

The significant changes that confront people in later life are successfully overcome by those who are flexible and willing to change. Indeed, it may be necessary to discard familiar activities and habits, and to replace them with new ones. At the same time it is important for people to retain their identity. Submitting to the pressures of a society which undervalues its older citizens can only have a negative outcome.

Interpersonal Relationships

Involvement with other people is important to the maintenance of mental health. Withdrawal from society, introspection and negative self-talk can lead to isolation and loneliness. The happy times in life may be enriched by sharing them with family and friends, while at times of sadness or crisis the support from others is invaluable. Love, anger and frustration are only a few of the many feelings experienced when interacting with other people. They provide variety, colour and intensity to life.

Self-respect

Pride in past achievements, high self-esteem and a feeling of being a worthy individual are all positive attributes that promote a feeling of wellbeing. Maintaining previous standards of dress and behaviour are simple but important ways of retaining pride in oneself. Helping family, friends or society in general may add purpose to life. For people who are not content with retirement, starting a new career may be necessary to retain a sense of self-worth.

ADJUSTING TO CHANGE

A person's status and standing in society is frequently determined by their occupational achievements, economic prosperity and role as a parent. Some of these values are not relevant to older individuals who may have retired from work, be living on a fixed income and who have already raised their children. As a result they may feel less valuable to the community and have a negative self-image. We will turn now to some specific events and issues which arise later in life, and consider ways these may be met and overcome successfully.

Retirement

'Retirement is retirement from full-time employment, not retirement from life.' It is an important event which reflects the community's belief that it marks the transition from middle to old age. Retirement has become a rite of passage, on a par with other important events such as christenings, barmitzvahs and weddings. This concept is rapidly becoming outdated, however, as many people elect to retire earlier, as young as fifty-five. It is therefore incorrect to view retirement as the beginning of 'old age'. At age sixty men, on average, can expect to live another fourteen years, while women may live a further twenty years. Retirement can represent a quarter of a lifetime, certainly a significant proportion that should be valued and enjoyed. In the past, later life was approached negatively, but this antiquated idea is rapidly changing. In the future retirement will be viewed as a new and exciting time.

The work ethic is a powerful force in our society. Work is viewed not only as a source of income, but can be the focus of many people's lives. An occupation may reflect status in the community and shape self-image and identity. Social relationships and friendships are other important benefits that flow from interactions with people at work. It is hardly surprising then, that retirement can significantly affect a person's way of life.

The Stages of Retirement

Although the physical act of retirement occurs abruptly, the adjustment starts some time before and proceeds through a number of phases until a new role and attitude has evolved and been accepted. Figure 2.1 demonstrates the six stages, two before and four after retirement, through which many people progress. It illustrates the commonly experienced feelings that relate to this period of transition, but is not a rigid plan to which everyone strictly adheres.

Thinking and planning for retirement usually begins many years beforehand. At this early *pre-retirement* time there may be a winding down of work, as well as financial planning for the future. Retirement is viewed as a positive event, but because of its remoteness in time is still in the realms of unreality. As the time to leave work approaches, the finality of this imminent major life event hits home, and it may be viewed negatively. This change usually occurs immediately before retirement, as feelings of insecurity and uncertainty about the future arise.

After retirement comes a *fantasy* period in which there is a feeling of euphoria, of being on a perpetual holiday and free to pursue interests previously denied by the constraints of work. For those who have planned well for retirement, enjoy good health and have financial security, this phase is prolonged, and gradually merges into a pleasant daily routine. For many others, however, this positive and exciting experience is followed by a period of *disenchantment*. This disappointment may be due to unrealistic expectations of later life — a holiday cannot continue forever. Other problems may arise if only short term goals are planned. After returning from a well-planned world trip, for instance, day-to-day life may seem empty and unsatisfying. Alternatively, planned activities may not turn out to be as fulfilling as expected, and boredom may become a problem. It then becomes necessary to re-examine the situation and make some modifications. A more realistic assessment of life after retirement occurs during this period of *reorientation*, new activities are explored and new goals are set. The implementation of these plans leads to a more permanent and positive attitude. Once these changes have been incorporated into the daily routine, *stability* returns. The retiree has accepted her or his new role.

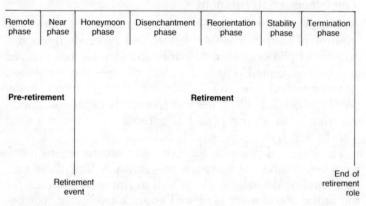

FIGURE 2.1 The stages of retirement.

Practical Considerations

The most obvious change is the increase in *free time*. The daily ritual of work is replaced by an unstructured day. While working, weekends and holidays are cherished, but, surprisingly, on retirement this flood of time can be disconcerting. Although most people initially enjoy this freedom, they soon seek to structure and timetable their days. Indeed, after a period of adjustment many people comment that they are so busy that they cannot understand when they found the time to work!

More time is spent at *home*, usually in the company of a spouse. The impact of retirement on a marriage varies, but generally is a reflection of the previous marital relationship. If the couple functioned well because they relied on distance in their relationship, then in retirement this lifestyle is best continued. Other couples become closer when they spend extra time together. Married couples develop a new equilibrium after a period of adjustment. Maintaining involvement with other people including neighbours, family and friends is an important factor in an enjoyable later life. This social interaction prevents the isolation and loneliness that can lead to a negative cycle of events and finally illness or dependency.

Increased *leisure time* means that people are able to begin new activities or pursue activities participated in before retirement more fully. Developing hobbies, taking part in sport and pursuing other interests in preparation for retirement ensures a smoother transition. A new balance is established with less time devoted to work or career interests and a greater emphasis on leisure.

> After Bill retired eighteen months ago we argued a lot. I still had my housework to do and he always seemed to be in the way. Now that he helps with the housework and has a part time job, I enjoy the extra time we have together. With Bill not working there is also more time to visit our daughter and grandchildren in Canberra.
>
> Joy (65)

Another important consideration in retirement is an adequate *income*. Financial security is necessary in order to take full advantage of leisure time, and to maintain an established lifestyle. On retirement income and assets are usually fixed, so careful planning is necessary. Accommodation and housing are also affected by income. For an enjoyable and self-sufficient later life accommodation should meet an individual's current needs, and be of their own choosing.

The relationship between retirement and *health* has been extensively studied. People in high pressure jobs feel blessed relief and suffer from fewer stress related illnesses when they are freed from the strain of their work. Although early retirement can be due to ill health, retirement itself is not associated with an increased incidence of illness. In fact evidence suggests that it can result in an improvement in physical and mental health, because there is more time to concentrate on recreational activities, exercising and eating a balanced diet. Good physical and emotional health contribute to an enjoyable life at any age.

Society's view of the elderly and an individual's own *self-image* change on retirement. The old negative stereotypes are slowly being replaced by a more realistic view of later life. A new career in retirement may involve part-time paid or voluntary work, creative hobbies, gardening or further education. Adopting a positive new role in retirement ensures the continuation of a fulfilling and active life. If older individuals view themselves in a positive way the wider community will also adopt a more positive attitude towards retirement.

Planning a Successful Retirement

Although retirement is significant and often stressful, the majority of people are able to cope with this change. Research has revealed that over two thirds of retirees adjust well to retirement. Of course the strategies for coping vary between individuals — there is no single approach for all people. Some simply relax and passively accept the changes, while others are busy with a full schedule of organized activities. The final group are those who enjoy the increased amount of leisure time and use it to develop new interests. Many of them have in common a positive attitude to life, are independent and have high self-esteem. Usually they have retired voluntarily and been involved in choosing the appropriate time to leave work. Surprisingly, they often held jobs which they enjoyed, not working for money alone. In effect, these people were successful in enjoying their work and continue this attitude into retirement.

Planning for retirement should start at least five to ten years beforehand. It should include the consideration of a wide variety of topics ranging from finance, housing and health, to recreational activities. In addition the intangible issues, such as changes in attitude, emotional readjustment and personal relationships, should be dealt with to ensure a smooth transition. The interrelationship of these factors is demonstrated in Figure 2.2.

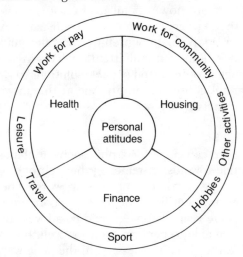

FIGURE 2.2 The interrelationship of tangible and intangible factors which affect a person on retirement.

Some people may wish to stay in full or part-time work. Consulting positions may be especially attractive, where the talents acquired over many years are utilized without the previous responsibilities and pressures. Other people are more adventurous, and broaden the possibilities to include a new job, retraining, further education or acquiring a new skill. Voluntary or community work are also areas that are keen to recruit people.

When I first retired the novelty of having nothing to do wore off quickly. Fortunately I had always enjoyed golf and it was good to be able to play more often. On most days after reading the paper in the morning I would think to myself 'What will I do now?' I started talking to other people and heard about Probus. My skills in running my own business are now used in my role as secretary of the local Probus*, a club for professional and business people which meets regularly and organizes activities.

Michael (67)

* Contact through the Rotary Club

Both partners should be involved in such planning, this can prevent future misunderstandings and arguments. Discussing the options with family and friends can also help clarify problems. There are now a number of organizations that arrange pre-retirement courses and these are listed in Appendix 2. In addition, individual counselling can offer guidance on the issues that require personal attention. This involves looking at the range of options and possible solutions to a problem, and after careful consideration arriving at the answer which best suits the individual's needs.

The Future

In the future we can hope for a philosophical change in the general attitude towards retirement, where chronological age will no longer be a criteria for ceasing work. There is no logical reason or scientific evidence to support retirement at sixty to sixty-five years. People should be allowed to work as long as they are able to perform their job well, but permitted to retire when they find it necessary. In the same way, if older people become unemployed, then their age should not be a barrier to new employment or retraining in another field of endeavour.

The preparation for retirement could be partly sponsored by a person's employer. After many years of valuable service there is some shared responsibility, by the employer and by society more generally, to help in the preparation for this next phase of life. Wider involvement in retirement issues is potentially valuable and educative for all concerned. It is steps like this which can contribute to the breaking down of negative stereotypes in the community, and ensure a fulfilling later life for older people.

Housing

A comfortable place to live significantly influences the quality of life. A home may not only be a treasured possession because of convenient modern appliances, but also because it harbours a host of fond memories. The neighbourhood is also well known, with its familiar shops, church and local doctor. Lifetime friendships with neighbours are a strong bond with the area. Most importantly the home is an individual's own domain, a symbol of independence and dignity.

In later life many aspects of a home which were initially desirable may become disadvantageous. As a result of children having left home, or economic and health factors, accommodation requirements may need to be reconsidered. The house may be too large, the maintenance beyond a person's capabilities, or better public transport and community facilities may be required. These are the sorts of issues often raised by family and friends. Other people's advice is usually well-intentioned, but occasionally the motives can be selfish. Although it is most important to listen to the spectrum of advice offered, the final decision must rest with the person making the move.

The wide variety of choices in accommodation reflect the diversity of people's needs and desires. This can range from moving interstate to a warmer climate for an active outdoor lifestyle, to nursing home accommodation required by the dependent and frail. At any age moving is a traumatic event and this remains the case in later life, particularly if it is the result of unfortunate circumstances such as illness or bereavement. The following discussion should serve as a guide for those faced with this crucial decision and ensure that all the alternatives have been considered so that the best decision is made.

Staying at Home

Most Australians over sixty remain in their own homes (93 per cent) and the first decision is whether an older person should even consider moving. The familiarity of the neighbourhood, the local shops, transport and community facilities are obvious inducements to remain. This is not to deny that moving is one possible answer to the problems that may arise. One approach is to consider solutions to problems that do not involve moving to a different area. To achieve this may involve seeking support from family, friends and outside agencies.

Staying at Home with Support

There are now available a number of government and community services that enable independent living in circumstances such as ill health and frailty. Visits from a home nursing service, for example, enable an earlier return from hospital to the home environment. Continued support allows chronically ill people to remain at home, receiving help in areas where they are having difficulty.

People may also consider moving because they can no longer perform the physical chores necessary to maintain a home. Here too referral to the correct agency may overcome the problem. House cleaning and maintenance can be carried out by the local council's home help and handyperson services, while occasionally an obliging neighbour may also be willing to offer assistance. A number of retired men are glad to mow lawns and undertake other odd jobs for friends and neighbours. Although this help may be volunteered without asking, there is no reason for those who require assistance not to request it.

> My main fear after the stroke was that I would have to go to a nursing home. For the first few days I could not move my left arm and leg, but gradually this has improved. I can now walk with a stick. The hospital arranged for rails to be fitted to the stairs, and a few other helpful modifications to the bathroom and kitchen so that I could return home. After leaving hospital my house always seemed to be busy. The nurse called for the first few weeks, and I also had the council's home help and meals on wheels. Now I can do most things for myself, although my grandson still comes to do the garden.
>
> Joan (76)

The family's anxiety and inability to sustain continuous care are often the triggers that result in moving. Many relatives are apprehensive when an older person lives alone and fear they may be unable to call for assistance in an emergency. If a house is big, taking in a boarder will allay this fear as well as provide companionship and support. A neighbour may also agree to check daily if necessary. Alternatively, small portable alarms are available. These can be carried and activated should an accident occur. Although this service may never be used, it both allays relatives' anxiety and the older person can continue to live independently in safety.

Moving to a Smaller House

Another option is to shift to a smaller home, perhaps remaining in the same area. If it is financially feasible, retaining the previous home and not selling until happily settled into the new accomodation is advisable. This enables flexibility for people who change their mind — occasionally the reality can differ from expectations.

Living with Family

Living with family, although not as common an occurrence in Australia as other countries, is also an alternative that warrants consideration. It is important to consider fully all the implications before proceeding with this move. Is there enough room and are all members of the family in agreement with the new arrangements? Different generations have different lifestyles. The noise and activity of a growing teenage family contrasts sharply with the tranquility of living alone. Privacy for all concerned is also important and must be safeguarded. Wishing to have 'time out' is a normal human emotion. A 'granny flat' on the same property is a compromise that can offer the benefits of proximity to the family while retaining each party's privacy.

> After mother fell and broke her hip she seemed to become weak and frail. I became concerned at her living alone, particularly as she was a long way from us. After some persuasion we reached a compromise and she agreed to move into a granny flat. It was a pleasant surprise to find the government would help to build it*. When we are on holidays mother spends time in the local hospital which has a respite-care programme.
>
> Jill (58)

The burden of responsibility may become too great for the relative who has taken on the role of caring. Although the obvious solution is to share responsibility with other family members this sometimes does not occur. A number of facilities are now available that offer either daily care with the person returning home in the evening, or respite care for a few weeks of the year. This support enables an older person

* Available in Western Australia and Victoria

to remain in a home environment but minimizes the stress on the family caregiver.

Group Housing

Group housing involves a number of people pooling their financial resources and sharing a house. Abbeyfield housing is similar, but has been tailored to the special needs of the elderly. A group of seven to ten people live together, with each person having his or her own room and sharing areas such as the kitchen and lounge. Combined decisions are made for the mutual benefit of all the residents. If necessary a caretaker can be employed, but often people prefer to care for themselves and each other. This type of accomodation offers the companionship of friends and maintains independence while remaining integrated in the community. In the future more of this type of housing is likely to become available.

Retirement Villages

Retirement villages have become increasingly popular in recent years. These comprise groups of self-contained units with adjoining recreational and sporting facilities. Their advantages include living with people of a comparable age who have similar interests, surrounded by all the amenities required. When contemplating this type of accommodation it is worth considering that not everyone enjoys close communal living. The emphasis on recreation and relaxation would not suit those who wish to remain active in business. These complexes can also be far from family and friends. If this is the case ensure there is adequate transport, enabling these contacts to be continued. The financial arrangements vary between different organizations and it is important to fully understand them before making a final committment. Many of these complexes are luxurious and therefore expensive. The Americanism 'woopies', well-off old people, has been coined to describe the wealthy group of retired individuals who can afford such accommodation.

Institutional Care

In certain circumstances the needs of some elderly, especially the ill or frail, may be best served by moving to accommodation where they can be cared for. Again, the overriding consideration must be that the person concerned retains control in making the decision where he or she will live. *Hostels* offer private rooms, often with facilities, and provide meals in a communal dining room. Although a person may be on-call in case of an emergency, generally the staff are not specially trained, so the residents must be fairly independent — they must be mobile and have control over their bodily functions. A number of hostels offer assistance to those who are dependent on others for some of their daily needs, such as bathing and dressing. Hostels offer a secure and comfortable environment for people who cannot or do not wish to live on their own.

If more intensive care is required then a *nursing home* may be more suitable. These provide twenty-four-hour care by qualified personnel for residents who are dependent on help for many of their needs. In recent years there have been dramatic physical improvements and a refreshing change in attitudes towards nursing home residents. Activities are now offered on a regular basis and socializing is encouraged. Maintenance of dignity and individuality in this difficult position of dependency, and ensuring that the rights of the individual are preserved at all times, are the objectives of current nursing home care. Rehabilitation is also emphasized. There can be a wide variation in standards between different institutions, so it is imperative to thoroughly investigate a home before making a decision. In addition the patient should receive a thorough assessment by a doctor with a special interest in the elderly, or by a geriatric assessment team. Occasionally there are medical conditions that can be identified and treated, making an alternative type of accommodation more appropriate.

Eight years ago my wife Lorraine was diagnosed as having Alzheimer's disease. The last few years have been a difficult struggle. Six months ago the strain was too much and I needed help. My GP called in an assessment team from the local geriatric hospital. They immediately arranged for Lorraine to go to hospital to give me a break. She returned home for a short time until a permanent place became available. I was very lucky as she is now in a home specially designed for people with Alzheimer's. There are plenty of places for her to walk but she cannot wander off the grounds. She has been able to take some of her personal things which helps her feel at home. Activities are also arranged almost every day and she can come out with me whenever I like.

Ron (76)

Making the Decision

There is often not a perfect solution to the question of accommodation. Each option has both advantages and drawbacks, with the final decision being a balanced compromise. Discussing the problem with friends and relatives can help to clarify the situation, and people who have already faced this dilemma can be a valuable source of information. Specialist advice is also available. Geriatric assessment teams are comprised of doctors, social workers and nurses who are used to dealing with such problems and can offer a professional, unbiased opinion.

Conflicting and confusing emotions are commonly experienced when a move is being considered. Loneliness, for instance, often motivates people to leave the family home. Helpful alternatives are sometimes seen as 'charity', and this misconception only limits the number of available options. Fear of becoming a burden on the relatives who offer to accommodate an older person in their home is also common. Discuss these feelings openly as they are often irrational and without foundation. Failure to do so may result in excellent suggestions being ignored, and the final decision being unsuitable.

The physical environment is an obvious starting point for an assessment. The accommodation must be attractive and inviting. It should be large enough for an individual's needs and personal belongings, but compact enough to ensure low maintenance. Public transport, shops and community facilities are important considerations, as these amenities enable an independent lifestyle. Proximity to friends, relatives and clubs, either in the same locality or by public transport, is essential if friendships and contacts are to be maintained.

Visiting the various types of accommodation provides personal knowledge and ensures the individual is involved in the final decision. Talk to the present residents to determine if they are pleased with the standard of care and accommodation provided. Check on the provision of adequate privacy and if personal freedoms are respected. Cherished personal possessions are difficult to part with, so inquire whether these can be brought into the new accommodation. The attitude and friendliness of the staff influences the atmosphere in which the residents live. There is usually a general feeling and impression obtained from these visits. Is the feeling one of living in a sterile institution or a friendly home? Trust these instincts as well as objectively evaluating the situation.

The financial arrangements should also be considered at this stage. Some people hesitate to ask, feeling it is impolite or not relevant until a decision has been made. Many accommodation villages and homes are run as a business and should welcome such inquiries. If the details seem too complex then seek professional advice. If possible ensure the decision is reversible by suggesting living in the new environment for a 'trial period'. As mentioned earlier, it is sometimes worth retaining the previous home, if possible, to allow for any change of mind should the new accommodation prove unsuitable. After considering all the alternatives discussed above, it is imperative that the final decision rests with the individual making the move.

A period of readjustment follows any move, and if this has been preceded by ill health or bereavement the problems may be compounded. There is usually a grief reaction to the loss of familiar surroundings and parting with past memories. Support from friends and relatives can facilitate a smooth transition.

Relationships

Although the emphasis has been on independence, this does not imply that a person should live in isolation. Interaction with other people is important for socializing and communication. It is often beneficial to share ideas or emotions with a confidant, and the burden of making decisions is eased if there is someone with whom we can discuss problems. Happy experiences are enhanced by enjoying them with others, while support from friends eases the distress of sadness and grief. Not only do relationships provide an opportunity for social involvement, they also bolster self-esteem and add purpose to life.

The majority of people in later life maintain frequent contact with family, friends and neighbours, and are involved in a variety of activities. Although the pattern of relationships tends to follow those established in earlier years, all personal interactions are dynamic and alter in response to the changes that occur throughout life. Those who anticipate and adjust to changing relationships are more likely to age successfully.

Marriage

The stability and security of marriage can act as a buffer against the many changes that occur in later life, and there is evidence that married men live longer than their unmarried counterparts. Most couples rely on each other for practical as well as emotional support, feeling comfortable and secure with a caring lifetime companion. Marriages invariably alter as the couple respond and adapt to the many changes that take place. Retirement and children leaving the family home provides an opportunity for intimacy and a greater sharing of interests and activities, for example. Some relationships strengthen as a result of these changes while others cannot tolerate this closeness. The cliché 'I married him for better and worse but not for lunch' summarizes what some women feel when their husbands retire. Each relationship will establish a new equilibrium that suits the particular couple.

The adjustments which occur within a marriage in response to the changes in later life include the sharing of domestic work if this was previously done by only one partner. The marriage thus becomes more 'equal'. Women tend to become more assertive while husbands communicate and share more of their feelings. If a partner becomes ill it is usually the spouse who cares for her or him. A person will probably feel most secure when being cared for by a loyal and loving companion.

In addition to time spent together it is advisable to foster interests and friendships outside the marriage. This allows a variety of different relationships to develop and prevents the boredom that can arise from being in a constant relationship. In the event of the death of a spouse a network of other friends has been established which may ease the grief and loneliness. As has been mentioned, women tend to live longer

than their husbands, and they rely on friendships to cope with
this crisis. On the other hand, statistics reveal that if a man
is widowed he will usually remarry.

There are one third more women than men over the age
of sixty-five and this makes it easier for widowers to find a
partner. Most are motivated by the happy experiences of their
previous marriage, seeking companionship and a similar
relationship with their new partner. There are a number of
pitfalls in choosing a companion at this time of life. In order
to erase the distress of loneliness and grief a hasty marriage
to a person who is incompatible may occur. Practical details
such as where to live and financial arrangements may not be
discussed because they are considered 'unromantic'. This can
lead to misunderstandings and conflict. A retired married
couple frequently spend more time together, and this can
highlight differences. It is necessary to consider such things
carefully before making a final decision.

The Family

It is sometimes thought that because the small nuclear family
has become the focus of family life, older people are excluded
and abandoned by their relatives. This is not usually the case.
While few older parents now live in the same house with
their adult 'children', the present structure of the *extended
family* involves a web of interdependent households connected
by the strong bonds of kindship and affection. This extended
family is larger than in previous times due to people living
longer. Most older people retain a close relationship with
other members of their family, even if distance limits this to
communicating only by phone. Remaining involved in family
affairs offers a special opportunity to interact with relatives
of various ages.

Support provided by the different generations within the
family is usually mutually beneficial. It is often the older members who are a source of both practical and emotional support
to families striving to cope with the stresses of work and growing children. This assistance can range from babysitting to
helping financially during periods of economic hardship. Pen-
sions have removed the onus on children to financially
subsidize their parents who may no longer be working. Often,
in fact, the opposite is now true, with children receiving

economic assistance from parents. Emotional support, especially as a result of marital conflict and divorce, is also an increasingly common occurrence, and it is frequently the parents on whom the younger generation rely for assistance during these times. On the other hand it is usually the adult children who care for their elderly parents during periods of ill health, and accept the responsibility of long term care if this becomes necessary.

Grandparenthood

A unique relationship in later life is that of grandparenthood. It was only relatively recently, again as the result of a healthier and longer life, that grandparents gained prominence in the extended family. The majority enjoy the role and become involved with their grandchildren, although sometimes work or geographical distance mean that the opportunities to develop a close relationship are limited.

Grandparents are often overcome with feelings of fulfilment, joy and love towards their grandchildren. There is usually more time to savour this experience, free from work and other responsibilities that were present when their own children were a similar age. The grandparent-grandchild relationship is an emotional bond based on companionship and love. The grandparent is generally not an authoritarian figure in the child's life, and so is not burdened by the responsibility of child-rearing. Having said this, it is important that grandparents do not usurp parents' authority. This can only create unnecessary tension within the family.

Grandparents are often the first people outside the nuclear family to accept and relate to children, encouraging them to establish their own identity separate from parents and siblings. Often grandchildren are at a pre-school age when grandparents are young and energetic. The bond is especially strong at this time and their love is returned unconditionally. During adolescence children usually become more independent, and although they may not visit their grandparents as frequently, may remain emotionally close.

I enjoy spoiling the grandchildren. It seems to me that I have the best of both worlds, as I play with them when they are happy and can give them back to their mother if they become upset.

My only regret is that I missed this time with my own children because of work.

Stan (68)

Overcoming and coping with the challenges of later life offers a positive model to the younger generation. Remaining active, involved and alert successfully negates the false stereotype of later life held by the wider community. Grandparents may also provide invaluable help during times of crisis. Because they are generally regarded as impartial, they may be able to mediate between parents and teenage children, for example. As mentioned, their help may also be needed during times of crisis such as divorce. Maternal grandparents are generally more involved here, due to the present trends in child custody. The situation can be quite complex, for instance when a divorced son or daughter remarries and establishes a second family. Losing contact with grandchildren following divorce, misunderstandings or geographical separation is a distressing and painful experience. The recently established Grandparents Support Group (see Appendix 2) is a self-help group that assists those who have lost contact with their grandchildren.

Aiding children who are homeless or uncared for by their parents is another area where older people can be immensely helpful. The Foster Grandparent Scheme is designed to be mutually beneficial, and matches an older person with a child who has a disability. The child receives affection and understanding, while the 'special grandparent' feels that their help is of great value.

Parents and Adult 'Children'

A normal parent-child relationship gradually changes to one of adults interacting as equals, and this new equilibrium may be preceded by a power struggle as the young generation exercises its newly acquired independence. Different lifestyles and values are potential sources of conflict. Choosing not to have children, living in a de facto relationship and the increasing frequency of divorce have only relatively recently become commonplace. They may remain foreign and a source of distress to parents regardless of their 'children's' age.

Interestingly, the 'generation gap' is less marked within families than in the wider community. This is partly due to the influence of family values and expectations permeating through the different generations. Ethnic and religious beliefs are also important factors that bond families and maintain traditional values.

The Role of Carer

In the event of disease, incapacity or terminal illness, one member of the family usually takes on the responsibility of care. In most instances it is a female, either the wife who tends to be healthier and live longer than her husband, or the middle-aged daughter, caring for her parents or parents-in-law. The motivation for caring can range from love to feelings of commitment and obligation. It can be a means of repayment for past favours. Knowing that institutional care is the only alternative may also compel a reluctant family to accept the care of their ill and frail relative. Frequently it is a combination of all these things that motivates a family to take on the responsibility of home care.

There is increasing recognition that these caregivers themselves need support, as they cope with the normal stresses of modern living as well as a dependent person. They make up a section of the community whose voluntary work is taken for granted. The devotion of some caregivers can reach a point where it jeopordizes their own health and happiness. Physical ailments such as backache, arthritis and high blood pressure are commonly related to physical and mental stress. Caregivers also frequently suffer from exhaustion, feeling emotionally drained, depressed and anxious. Some of this is undoubtedly the result of trying to fulfill responsibilities to both the dependent person and towards one's own family and work — the load is simply too much. Needless to say, the strain may spill over to negatively affect family relationships, and there are fewer opportunities for social contact, with little time for leisure and friendships. Loss of income as a result of leaving work to care for a dependent person can add financial hardship to an already stressed family. The government offers a small allowance in certain circumstances and those who are eligible should apply.

Negative thoughts and feelings are often suppressed for fear that voicing concerns may be interpreted as being unfaithful and complaining about a loved one. Even when help is available the caregiver may not accept it, viewing this as an admission of failure to provide adequate care. Other people are possessive and not willing to relinquish this responsibility, sincerely believing that they are the best person to look after their own family member.

I started to get headaches and could not sleep at night even though I was physically exhausted. The doctor told me it was overwork from looking after mother who has dementia. He arranged for mother to go to hospital for a week and suggested relaxation classes or yoga. That was the turning point, when I realized that at the pace I was going mother would outlive me! I learnt to be stronger and insisted that she attend a group for the 'elderly confused', twice each week. This gave me more time for other work, my family and a game of tennis once a week. The health centre also suggested that I contact ADARDS* who have been very helpful. The most difficult job was to convince my brother to look after mother every few weekends. Life is quite good now and with time to do the things I enjoy, I don't resent looking after mother.

Leila

The ability of carers to cope is often determined by the amount of assistance they receive. This can be in the form of emotional support, financial aid, or encouragement and recognition of their work by family and friends. At different times all of these forms of help may be required. It is important that equal consideration be given to the needs and wishes of both the dependent person and the relative providing the care. The carer should be determined to maintain previous interests and an enjoyable lifestyle. Unfortunately caregivers may sacrifice these pleasures; this can rapidly lead to exhaustion, resentment and an inability to cope. A positive attitude depends on the carer maintaining his or her own health and wellbeing, as well as recognizing the limits of his or her abilities. Extra help should be sought, or a holiday or break from the daily routine arranged, before these limits are exceeded.

* Alzheimer's Disease and Related Disorders Society

Support groups can also lighten the burden often felt by caregivers. An important function of these groups is education. Understanding an illness can explain some of the problems encountered, and may influence planning for the future. The Alzheimer's Disease and Related Disorders Society [ADARDS] is an excellent example of a very successful self-help group whose aim is to inform and assist families of people who suffer from Alzheimer's disease. Such groups provide an opportunity to share personal experiences with those in a similar situation and help resolve problems that may arise. There is often a feeling of relief as carers realize that many of their difficulties and feelings are not unique. Community services such as 'home help', 'meals on wheels' and the home nursing service are also valuable resources that can be called on to ease the burden of home care.

As mentioned, it is essential for the carer to have time off — their work can sometimes occupy the full twenty-four hours in a day. This respite can take the form of regular day programmes, in which the dependent person attends an activity or discussion group on certain days of the week, returning home in the evening. It is advisable that the carer plan three to four rest periods each year, and during this time other family members may be able to take over the responsibility. If this is not possible an alternative is inpatient respite care. The ill or frail person is admitted to either hostel or nursing home accommodation, depending on their needs, and stays there for the duration of the carer's holiday.

Institutional care is often the last resort. A carer must recognize, however, that at some stage he or she may no longer be able to cope, or be able to provide the type of care needed. In this case a carer should not feel guilty; it is a reality which may have to be confronted.

There are a number of pitfalls to be avoided if a family is to take on the responsibility of providing for the needs of a dependent or ill person. It is stating the obvious to suggest that if people have not enjoyed a good relationship in the past, it is unwise to take on this role which involves closer and more frequent contact. Problems can also arise when anxious relatives underestimate the ability of a person to function alone, and suggest that they should live together in the same home, or the person move to communal accommodation. This is particularly common following bereavement or illness. Impulsive and incorrect decisions may be made as a result of stressful events, and these can be difficult to reverse. During traumatic periods, although support and understanding is needed, this should not go as far as placing a person in a dependent position, in which she or he may soon lose confidence and take on a passive role. If there is confusion or disagreement about the level of self-sufficiency, an impartial professional assessment can be arranged by a doctor.

Friendships

After retiring, what surprised me was how quickly I lost touch with friends at work. Whenever I met them I felt left out as they always were talking about what was happening at work. Before long I stopped visiting my old work mates. My wife, as always, continued her own busy schedule and I began to feel lonely. Until then I had always considered bowls for old people but decided to try it when a neighbour invited me. I was pleasantly surprised to find many people of my own age, and I have become friendly with a whole new group of warm and welcoming people.

Jeff (69)

Friends provide a necessary and valuable contribution to people's lives at all ages. Friendships may thrive and develop, sometimes becoming closer than family relationships. Devotion and approval from friends improves a person's confidence and morale. At times of stress confidants can provide support and consolation, alleviating the burden of suffering. Sharing experiences with a companion also adds to the enjoyment of happy occasions. In short, friendships encourage continued social contact which prevents physical and mental isolation. For many people friendships are established in the workplace. On retirement, however, these friendships may fall away. In anticipation of this, it is important that people establish relationships outside work before retirement. This is particularly important for men, who generally do not form intimate friendships as women do, and for people who have not married or who have not had children. Clubs and organisations offer the opportunity to be involved in social and sporting activities, and are excellent venues for meeting people.

Not surprisingly there is often a similarity of age, background and interests among friends. The present trend to separate older people from the rest of the society by establishing retirement villages is based on the belief they provide all the activities and facilities that are needed. Initiating and maintaining friendships is certainly easier in these communities, and therefore loneliness is less common. However, the isolation can restrict contact with people who have different or fresh ideas, and of course it is desirable to interact with people of all ages. A close friendship with at least one young person is stimulating and keeps an older person in touch with current trends. In return a younger person can benefit from the wisdom and experience of an older person. The result is a mutually beneficial friendship, and improved communication and understanding between the generations.

Loneliness

Loneliness differs from being physically alone. It implies feelings of emptiness, boredom and worthlessness. There is an absence of intimacy, and no opportunity to share emotions or experiences. Of course many people enjoy solitude, or are mentally occupied so that they do not feel lonely. Most people, however, prefer to combine time alone with social and emotional involvement with friends and family.

We discussed the false negative stereotype that many older people are lonely in Chapter 1. Research has revealed that adolescence is the loneliest time of life and that this decreases with age. Most older people are not lonely. They lead full, active social lives and enjoy meaningful relationships with a number of other people. There is also great diversity in the range of personal contacts, which include family, friends and neighbours. The main contact tends to be with family, in particular one's own children.

Many activities remain centred around married couples. This disadvantages those who have suffered the loss of their spouse. Widows, who tend to have a closer network of friends, usually cope better with this problem than their male counterparts. Men, in particular, may suffer the dual loss of their spouse and retirement from work. They are often lonely and may remarry to combat this.

After Nola died my life was empty. We had always done everything together and the loneliness was unbearable. I could not
stay in the house alone and visited people till late at night. Coming home was the worst. Sally from across the road has been very
kind. She went through the same thing when she lost her husband two years ago. I am happy to have her companionship but
as we live so close there is no reason at the moment to get
married.

Jim (73)

Loneliness can lead to a decline in physical and emotional
health. A lonely individual loses interest in life, lacks mental
stimulation and participates in few recreational activities. He
or she may not exercise and often nutrition is poor. These
factors all compound the problem of ill health. The distress
of loneliness is believed to suppress the immune system which,
as we have seen, is responsible for protecting the body against
outside infections, plus the surveillance and destruction of
cancer cells. As a result there is often an increased incidence
of disease among lonely people. Poor health itself can cause
social isolation. Those who are blind, deaf or disabled have
a greater risk of becoming isolated and lonely. They require
special attention and added support to remain active, participating members of society.

Loneliness can be overcome, but like all worthwhile endeavours it requires effort and determination. Loneliness is
usually the result of a number of losses. These often include
retirement (less contact with workmates), and the death of a
friend or spouse. Taking tranquillizers in order to alleviate
the feelings of emptiness and boredom is not the solution. It
is preferable to fill this vacuum by socializing, becoming involved with other people and participating in activities.
Seeking out those with similar interests and initiating new
friendships will prevent loneliness. The skill of listening to
other people's opinions and being tolerant of their points of
view will encourage friendships to grow. If romance evolves
it will add intimacy and affection to the relationship.

The family usually remains the most important source of
support and company. Visits are encouraged by being warm
and hospitable. If people are made to feel guilty for not coming more often, the visits become unenjoyable and less

frequent. Remaining involved in family matters also sustains these relationships. Neighbours are often more important in later life, as they may be the only practical friendships available due to limitations of health and transport. It is important to keep this in mind when contemplating a move. Those with pets are also less lonely. The companionship and affection offered by an animal, who in turn relies on its owner for all its needs, can provide many hours of enjoyment.

Planning is also important in combating loneliness. Often it is the evenings and on weekends that these unpleasant feelings are most intense. Loneliness can be alleviated by being occupied at these times, with valuable and rewarding activities. This may include sports, or intellectual pursuits such as further education. It may also be helping others in need, visiting friends and relations, working at a craft, taking up a new hobby — the list is endless. Loneliness is *not* a normal part of later life.

Special Considerations for Women

Older women suffer the double prejudices of sex and age discrimination (sexism and ageism). They constitute a significant proportion of the community but their low profile results in many of their particular needs being ignored. There is an abundance of advice on retirement, a principally male-dominated event, but little consideration to the effect of ageing on women who continue to lead a traditional life in the home. For these women the transition of later life is less abrupt than retirement. Their work at home proceeds uninterrupted, with their daily routine remaining clearly defined and unchanged. On the other hand, children leaving the family home is more keenly felt by the mother, and causes her to re-evaluate the future. The feeling of no longer being needed by grown family members is sometimes termed the 'empty nest' syndrome. In addition it is usually a women who cares for elderly relatives. This can result in a conflict between the responsibilities she feels towards her husband, children and grandchildren, and the dependent person. A network of friendships is often well established, and these can be important in helping her overcome such problems.

As we have seen, women have an increased life expectancy, outliving men by about five years. This fact, and the tendency among women to choose older partners, results in a period of widowhood of approximately ten years. Indeed, widowhood is so prevalent in later life that it could be considered a normal life cycle event. The traumatic crisis that follows the death of a spouse is usually more distressing than previous events in a woman's life. Fortunately most women adjust to this loss and after a time gain a new stability. Good health and financial security are also valuable in easing the burden of grief and ensuring a satisfactory adjustment to new circumstances. In the future a greater number of women will be financially secure and independent, and this change is likely to ease the plight of older women. A change in societal expectations may also see women marrying younger men. As a result a woman will be less likely to outlive her partner. The numerical strength and political awakening of older women is likely to ensure that the issues relevant to them will not be ignored, but dealt with by politicians who are always sensitive to new electoral pressures.

Health

Good health is central to the enjoyment of later life and an individual's independence. Illness limits the ability to continue working, and can have a detrimental effect on mobility, choice of accommodation and self-sufficiency. The emotional consequences of ill health may not only diminish the general feeling of wellbeing, but can result in fear and depression. There is no doubt that the incidence of illness increases with advancing age, but the image of older people as ill invalids is excessively pessimistic. A survey of those aged over sixty years revealed that two thirds enjoy good health, with only 14 per cent reporting poor health. Most of the illnesses are fortunately minor. During periods of stress and transition, such as retirement and bereavement, people are more vulnerable to disease. In addition illness may have a greater impact on an older person's life, with incomplete recovery a more frequent occurrence. Health is therefore an important issue that must be tackled both from the point of view of preventing disease, as well as suggesting ways of coping and adjusting to illnesses that may arise.

Ageing does not cause any of the diseases that occur in later life. As we emphasized earlier, it is not 'normal' for an older person to feel ill. Many of the illnesses which occur later in life begin with mild symptoms such as tiredness or weakness which, because they are not disabling, lead a person to accept them as part and parcel of ageing. Often, because of this false belief, an older person will endure far more discomfort and inconvenience than when he or she was younger. Symptoms that should alert a person to a problem are frequently ignored, and the disease may progress unchecked for some time. Incontinence, for example, is often endured by older people — they may accept it as 'normal' and may also be embarrassed to discuss the problem. Poor vision and deafness are disabilities which are tolerated at no other time than in old age. In addition to the physical problems associated with the loss of these special senses, the emotional consequences may be profound, as communication with other people breaks down. Irrespective of age, all possible avenues should be explored to improve the sight and hearing, but if this is not possible assistance should still be sought to minimize any handicap.

Dad seemed to be forgetful and had difficulty concentrating. Many of the things he said were not relevant to the conversation. I thought it was the beginning of dementia. Also speaking to him on the phone was becoming impossible although he continued to deny he could not hear. Finally he agreed to see the doctor, and I was right, he needed a hearing aid. Dad is now more alert and interested in things. I realise a lot of the 'memory' problems were simply due to deafness.

Alice

A further complication is the fact that a number of diseases present in a different way later in life. The symptoms, therefore, may be ignored because they are not recognized as indicating disease. Heart disease can be present without chest pain, and the temperature is not always elevated with an infection. Fatigue and loss of appetite are more subjective feelings that should not be ignored if they persist. Emotional problems can manifest themselves in physical symptoms, making it difficult to decide if the problem is physical, mental or both.

An important measure of good health is a person's ability to go about their life normally. If there is an abrupt change this may indicate a problem is developing. For example, the sudden onset of breathlessness, or confusion in familiar surroundings, usually indicates a problem. Often it is a friend or relative who first becomes aware of these subtle changes. The cause may not always be obvious, in the case of confusion, for instance, the problem may be affecting the brain but originating elsewhere in the body. A full check-up is advisable as soon as symptoms appear; early diagnosis usually ensures a better response to treatment.

A positive approach should be adopted by both patients and doctors, and all relevant complaints should be explored, irrespective of age. Many conditions are able to be treated, or at least alleviated, resulting in an improved quality of life. Patience and optimism are needed since the recovery time can be longer than in previous years. In the case of incomplete recovery, an optimistic attitude must continue and rehabilitation should be commenced. There are also many diseases that require a person to have regular checkups. It is wise to have a local doctor so that contact can be maintained.

Coping with Illness

The onset of illness is a threatening experience. It is often accompanied by feelings of grief resulting from the loss of good health. Fear of death or of becoming dependent on others may also be experienced. The treatment itself may be stressful, especially if it is necessary to spend time in a hospital. In the latter situation, a sense of having lost control may arise, particularly where the decision-making is handed over to medical staff. Such feelings are frequently mixed with anger, guilt and depression.

It is a patient's right to be fully informed about a proposed treatment, and to know all the options available. Never feel too inhibited to ask questions, or voice an objection if there is a disagreement. It is important to express these feelings not only to medical staff but also to loved ones. These people are usually keen to offer support which may aid recovery. Talking about fears and worries eases the burden.

> I was devastated to discover a lump in my breast. The first doctor spoke 'down to me' as if it was not my body he was talking about. I insisted on a second opinion. The difference was amazing. Apparently there are a number of possible operations and all these were explained to me. I chose to have a breast reconstruction after the cancer was removed. The second doctor had my full confidence and respect.
>
> Christine (58)

It is often difficult to ask for help, but it may be necessary if complete independence is to be regained. Many people, of all ages, require assistance after an illness, or after having spent time in hospital. The help may be simply a stick for added stability while walking, or perhaps involvement in a rehabilitation programme. Many support groups are now established that can offer practical advice to assist patients and their families. Stroke, heart surgery and Parkinson's disease support groups are all active in major Australian cities. A patient should aim to resume a normal life by setting achievable goals. Attitude remains the most important factor for successfully adjusting and resuming a normal life. It is essential to retain a positive self-image — illness in no way decreases a person's worth.

Sexuality

Sexuality is an integral part of a healthy, happy and fulfilling life. It is a natural means by which people express love and affection. We looked at how older people are sometimes portrayed as asexual in Chapter 1, and at how this stereotype is not borne out by the facts. Our culture portrays beauty, youth and sexuality as inseparable. This is compounded in the assumption that with increasing age a person is physically and therefore sexually less attractive to the opposite sex. If these desires are present then a person may be viewed as sexually frustrated or even lecherous. Some older people come to regard their normal sexual feelings as shameful and embarrassing. It is crucial to change the prevailing stereotype, and for older people themselves not to fall victim to it.

Masters and Johnson, pioneers in researching human sexuality, concluded that the requirements for sex in later life were good health plus an interested and interesting partner. This positive view has been confirmed by studies which reveal that 70 per cent of elderly couples remain sexually active. This represents only a slight decline in sexual activity with age. Those who were most active sexually in their younger years continue this pattern of sexual activity into later life, while those who were never interested may use age as a convenient excuse to stop!

> As a young resident in hospital I recall discussing with a man in his eighties the need for removal of his testes to halt the spread of prostate cancer. To my surprise his main concern was that it put an end to his sex life. I hope after many years my attitude is now less prejudiced by preconceived ideas.
>
> Author

Sexual activity confirms that a person is attractive and desirable to the opposite sex, and reinforces that he or she is a 'sexual being'. This improves self-esteem and engenders a feeling of worth. Sex enhances relationships by providing another avenue through which to communicate feelings of affection. The closeness of physical contact, to be touched and caressed, is particularly important to those who may have impairment of other senses such as sight or hearing. In addition there is the excitement and release of sexual energies. Older people often have more time to enjoy sex, and many report an improvement in and greater enjoyment of sexual activity.

Ageing and Sex

Ageing causes definite biological changes to sexual function. These alterations do not detract from the enjoyment of sex, rather, they offer a different experience. Problems arise when these changes are misinterpreted as heralding the loss of sexual function. It is normal for an erection to be less firm in later life, for example, but if this is not known, it may be misinterpreted as a loss of libido. Subsequent sexual advances could then be rejected for fear of failure. We can see how easily problems can arise from social pressures and psychological inhibitions that are unrelated to ageing.

For men, it also takes longer for an erection to develop, so often more direct physical stimulation is required. The prolonging of sex not only ensures more pleasure and control, but is also less likely to result in premature ejaculation as is often the case with younger men. The ejaculation itself is usually less forceful and the amount of semen reduced. The erection then fades more rapidly and the time interval between repeated sex is longer (usually hours to days). As a result an ejaculation may not occur every time a man has intercourse.

The hormonal changes associated with menopause in women cause a number of symptoms including hot flushes and night sweats, but there is usually no significant reduction in sexual function. The vagina is often dryer and its lining thinner. These problems can be overcome by prolonging foreplay and maintaining regular sexual activity. If this is insufficient then hormone replacement therapy may be an option, or a vaginal lubricant can be used. Freedom from interruption by children and from the worries of contraception both contribute to increased sexual pleasure in older people.

The physiological changes discussed will invariably require a different approach to sex and a modification of expectations. Communication of pleasurable experiences and patience as each partner comes to terms and understands their new functions will result in a more satisfying relationship. An important means of maintaining sexual function is to continue sex regularly.

Illness and Sex

It is undeniable that illness affects sexual activity. Ill-health in either or both partners is commonly cited as the reason why sexual activity is ceased, and there are a number of diseases in which well-documented physical damage explains this decline. Diabetes can interfere with the ability of the nerve fibres to carry impulses to the genital organs, and this results in a loss of function. Hardening of the arteries (atherosclerosis) is often associated with smoking, and has recently been implicated in reducing blood flow to the penis, thus contributing to impotence. In addition a number of drugs, including certain blood pressure tablets and sedatives, have side effects that can interfere with normal sexual activity. These effects are rare, however, and the majority of people on such medications experience no problems. Any person who has a query regarding the effects of medication on sexual function should speak to their doctor.

Disease and surgery to the sex organs, is a more difficult and emotional issue. Hysterectomy or breast operations in women, and prostate surgery in men, can disturb sexual function. Although there is no physical connection between surgery to these organs and sexual performance, the operation may be interpreted as an assault on a person's sexuality. After mastectomy a women may avoid sexual intimacy as she feels self-conscious and unattractive. Support through this traumatic period, involving counselling both partners, in conjunction with reconstructive surgery or breast prosthesis, can help a women regain an active and satisfying sex life. Following prostate surgery in men, it is normal for semen to be deposited in the bladder instead of being expelled through the penis. Unnecessary anxiety will be prevented if he is aware that this is normal. Many myths contribute to these operations being associated with a decrease in sexual function. A person should fully understand the effects of the planned surgery. Counselling and reassurance regarding their sexuality afterwards will alleviate many of these problems.

Fear that sex could be harmful to health is common in people who have suffered a heart attack or stroke. The exertion required for intercourse is equivalent to climbing one to two flights of stairs, and therefore rarely needs to be avoided for reasons of health. It could in fact be argued that since exercise is encouraged after a heart attack, sex may be good for the heart. The risk of heart attack during intercourse is small, with a high percentage of these attributed to extramarital affairs. This suggests that unfaithfulness and *not* sex may be a major contribution factor!

The care in hospital was excellent. The details of the heart attack were explained in great detail. It was only when I arrived home that I realized nobody had spoken to me about sex. The booklet said it was OK to have intercourse after four weeks, but we decided to wait until the next appointment. The doctor explained that when I was able to do moderate exercise, equivalent to climbing a few flights of stairs, I could have sex. As we left his office I suggested to my wife we use the stairs rather than the lift!

Stan (68)

Arthritis is another common complaint which requires innovation and motivation to overcome the discomfort of painful joints. While making love new positions, perhaps using pillows for support, may be required. A warm bath to soothe the joints and even a pain relieving tablet beforehand contribute to minimizing the effect of arthritis on sexual enjoyment. If tiredness is a problem, love making can take place in the morning when the couple is rested.

Even in today's more enlightened society there remain a group of older people who continue to be denied their sexual freedom. The sexuality of those in long-term nursing and institutional care is not acknowledged and sexual expression is invariably prohibited. In the coming years one would hope that this denial of basic human emotions will be remedied.

Enjoying Sex

Sexual expression is extremely personal and the pleasure it provides does not diminish with age. It relieves sexual tensions and contributes to a feeling of 'wellbeing'. There are many aspects to sexual function, with intercourse being only one of these. The closeness of physical intimacy involving hugging, cuddling and caressing is equally important, and need not always lead to intercourse. There are many different sexual practices, all of which affirm a person's sexuality. These subjects have previously been taboo and some people may find it difficult to accept them as alternatives. They are, however, a fact of life and require consideration. The diversity in the way people express their sexuality reflects choices that suit individual desires and preferences.

Restriction due to a stroke or arthritis may limit a person's ability to have intercourse. This should not deny one the opportunity of sensual pleasure. Mutual masturbation often offers a practical solution. Stimulation of the penis, or breast and vaginal area culminating in an orgasm is one alternative. Occasionally aids such as vibrators can be used to increase the amount of stimulation, while oral sex is practised at all ages. A couple should work together to explore new and exciting sexual experiences that are mutually satisfying.

The reality of later life is that there are many single people, usually because their partner has died. We have seen that women tend to outlive men, so that there are more elderly women than men. Some older single people choose celibacy based on personal, moral or religious beliefs. Masturbation, as mentioned, is another alternative that satisfies sexual desires and reaffirms a person's sexuality. At all ages there are homosexual relationships, and later life is no exception. The wide spectrum of sexual activity confirms that age is not a barrier to many forms of sexual orientation and expression.

For a successful and satisfying sex life thought, effort and perseverence are required. Many problems can be avoided by sensible and often simple measures. Stress, tiredness and over-indulgence in food and alcohol are common causes for lack of sexual interest that can be easily remedied. Appearance and grooming are not only important in order to remain attractive to a partner but also to boost self-confidence. Sexual problems may stem from marital disharmony and it is important that a couple seek counselling if this is the case. Boredom with sex is a threat that should be tackled by experimenting with new ideas and different techniques. It is not too late to be innovative and explore untried alternatives. Communicating to a partner personal desires and pleasurable or exciting ideas is very important. In this way an active and satisfying sex life can be maintained into old age, free of social prejudice and personal inhibitions.

Death and Bereavement

Death is one of the few undeniable facts of life. It is an inevitable and natural way to complete the life cycle. Improved living conditions and advances in modern medicine have meant that death is no longer as accepted as it was in previous generations. Indeed, the denial of death has replaced sex as the taboo subject of modern times. The dying are hidden away or segregated in hospitals, and feelings of intense grief are often stifled under a disguise of stoic courage. With advancing age, the deaths of close friends and relatives force an older person to confront her or his own mortality. Facing death may result in a reappraisal of life. The realization that the future is finite may encourage an older person to discard unpleasant or irrelevant activities, and to replace them with others that bring joy and meaning to life. In this way the remaining years of life may be a person's fullest.

Death may evoke feelings of fear or denial. More commonly, however, the reality of human mortality is accepted. Changing circumstances may cause a modification of a person's attitude to death. It may be seen as a release from terminal illness, for example. It may also be viewed philosophically as the completion of a full and satisfying life.

Surprisingly, it is not death itself but the process of dying that causes people the most distress. The uncertainty of the future leads to a fear of what may be confronted while dying. Pain, loneliness, dependency and becoming a burden to loved ones are common causes of anxiety. Many outdated ideas on dying persist despite the revolutionary changes in the attitude and care of the terminally ill. The emphasis is now on the individual being informed and involved in the decisions regarding his or her care, and the ideal is to be in a caring and supportive environment. This may be at home with family who can receive help from visiting trained staff if necessary. The recent establishment of hospices means that the terminally ill can be comforted in the final stages of illness in a warm, caring environment. It is extremely important that the physical and psychological needs of an ill person are met so that they may die with dignity and without pain.

Coping with Death

In order to understand our own emotional reactions to death and cope with a terminally ill loved one, it is useful to know what is considered normal in the process of dying. Dr Elizabeth Kubler-Ross, a world authority on death and dying, has described five stages in a person's struggle to cope with death. These should not be viewed as progressive steps, as many people fluctuate between them and even miss different stages. Throughout the process of dying the hope of a remission or cure should be allowed to continue.

Denial The immediate reaction on being told one has a terminal illness is to deny that it is true. People commonly believe that they have been given the results of another patient by mistake. This protects them from reality, allowing time to psychologically prepare and cope with this devastating news. Gradually the truth is accepted, and gives rise to anger.

Anger The injustice that life is ending can lead to hostility and rage. Although this is often directed towards family and friends, the anger is in fact the surfacing of an internal emotional struggle with death. It is advisable to accept this as a normal reaction rather than strenuously defend oneself, as this may only increase the hostility. The anger usually subsides, giving way to bargaining.

Bargaining In a last attempt to change reality a person will try to bargain, usually with God, to prolong life in exchange for certain promises. When this fails, a person becomes depressed, as death is seen as inevitable.

Depression The illness has often progressed to the stage that its consequences are obvious. Depression is a normal human emotion in these tragic circumstances, and a person should be allowed to fully express these sentiments. At this time the support from friends and family is extremely important; they should be available to listen and share their feelings. In time the depression will gradually give way to a realization that death is unavoidable.

Acceptance An inner calm and serenity accompanies the acceptance of death. It is a time to be with family and loved ones, a time to say farewell. Coping with death is never easy, even when it is expected, but understanding that these intense emotions are normal allows us to cope better and offer support when it is needed.

Grief

Grief is the natural emotional response to a loss, applying in particular to bereavement. Older people usually experience a number of losses as they outlive their friends and relatives. The death of a loved one, especially a spouse, is an extremely distressing experience. Grief allows an outpouring of these intense emotions, enabling the person to eventually accept and adjust to their new circumstances. There is no quick or easy way to prevent this suffering. Although the outward display of grief may vary between different cultures, and may be influenced by the previous relationship with the deceased, there are a number of common emotions that are experienced by those grieving.

Immediately after being informed of the death most people are overwhelmed by an intense feeling of shock and disbelief. The news is bewildering and often denied. There is an expectation that the deceased will appear at any moment, even to the point of hearing her or his voice. This initial numbing of the emotions allows practical considerations, such as the funeral, to be arranged. This period of shock and bewilderment can last hours or days, but gradually gives way to the realization that a death has occurred, and that this cannot be altered.

Outbursts of crying, wailing and screaming are experienced as the impact of the loss hits home. Feelings that life is no longer worth living and expressing a wish to die are common. This sorrow can lead to depression and despair. Anger and guilt are also often experienced at this traumatic time. Anger may be directed at medical staff who are accused of neglecting to save the deceased, and even the dead person may be blamed for having caused this distressing event. Guilt related to past differences and arguments may be felt, as the grieving person reviews and comes to terms with the previous relationship. This time of intense distress and anguish may last for weeks or months, sometimes even years. Though these feelings gradually subside they may suddenly reappear, and cause a person to conclude that he or she may never recover from the loss. This is not the case, these lapses are a normal part of grieving.

Eventually the loss is fully accepted, and the mourner is able to face this reality. Feelings of sadness are less intense and positive emotions begin to reappear. A person has then 'let go' of previous emotional ties and is ready to seek alternative friendships and activities. A successful adjustment means more than simply seeking to replace the past, but aiming to establish a new and meaningful life for the future.

There is usually no fixed sequence to the events described above. They frequently overlap, and are experienced differently by many people. There is great individual variation in the duration and intensity of these feelings, but generally after one year most will have successfully accepted and coped with their loss. A resurgence of grief frequently occurs, particularly at important times such as anniversaries and birthdays. The intensity of these emotions usually subsides over subsequent years as a person becomes involved and finds fulfilment in a new life.

> I went to see my doctor about bad pains in the neck. He could find nothing seriously wrong and suggested it was most likely tension. We talked about how I was managing, and I told him that the worst seemed to be over. It was only after thinking about this at home that I realized the pain started a few days before the first anniversary of Bill's death.
>
> Lillian (81)

During mourning the bereaved have an increased risk of developing an illness. This is most prevalent in the first six months, and has usually abated after a year. Heart disease is the most common problem, the bereaved literally dying of a broken heart. Complicating this are the many physical symptoms experienced while grieving. These include chest pains, palpitations and stomach pains. If in doubt as to the nature of the complaints it is advisable to be thoroughly checked by a doctor. Successfully coping with grief will ensure that these problems are resolved.

Coping with Grief

The pain following the death of a loved one cannot be avoided. There are however a number of factors worth considering to ensure that the process of mourning is not prolonged or lead to unresolved psychological problems. It is advisable to view the dead body. This not only confirms beyond doubt the finality of the death, but offers an opportunity to say any last goodbyes. Rituals are also beneficial as they provide a framework for expressing emotions. The funeral is an opportunity to express grief. It verifies the death and brings together friends and relatives who are an important source of support for the mourners. Some cultures and religions restrict certain enjoyable activities or may advocate the wearing of particular clothing in recognition of the period of mourning. Another difficult but important milestone is the sorting out of the deceased possessions. It signifies that the reality of the death has been faced and a new life must start. All these events mark a progression through the normal grieving process and ensure that the death is coped with successfully.

Grief is best resolved by allowing painful and sad emotions to be expressed. This can be through crying or recounting past memories of the deceased, and working through the events leading up to her or his death. It is important to 'talk'. Some people may expect the mourner to 'keep a stiff upper lip' or advise him or her to 'snap out of it'. It is preferable, however, to trust one's intuition and allow these emotions to be expressed. Grief should not be suppressed or hurried. Drugs, such as tranquillizers and alcohol, do not resolve the burden and pain. Grief is a normal experience, not an illness that requires treatment. The feelings are temporarily numbed and suppressed by medication, but flood back when the effects of the drug have worn off.

Friends and relatives are an important source of support through these difficult times. Those who have suffered similar losses can offer comfort and hope based on their own experiences. Accept help from friends when it is offered, whether it is practical assistance such as transport, or friends simply being there for company. A person needs only one or a few close compassionate friends with whom to share grief. Those who are good listeners and show understanding are the most helpful. Immediately after the funeral many people are present to console the mourners, but some time later there is a common misconception that their support is no longer necessary. Those who are grieving may then feel deserted and alone.

Six weeks after Harry's death I expected to be feeling better. In fact I was getting worse; still not sleeping and no appetite for food. Most of my friends were busy with their own lives again. If it wasn't for a friend who was widowed two years ago I am not sure I would have come through those first six months.

Susan (71)

Maintaining independence and developing a daily routine is necessary to ensure a return to normal life. Although well-meaning friends may offer to shop and attend to other pressing needs, it is preferable for a person to resume these activities as soon as he or she feels ready — they allow a person to leave the house and interact normally with others. If a spouse dies the motivation for continuing activities previously done for the other person often goes. Food preparation is a good example here, and it is vital for this to be continued as nutrition is particularly important in times of stress. It is a challenge to develop new habits that take into account the changed circumstances. A person must consider her or himself a worthwhile individual, entitled to the same care and attention as previously.

Delaying or suppressing grief usually results in these powerful but unresolved emotions re-emerging in other, often destructive ways. Physical and emotional problems, commonly depression, develop in those who have not completely come to terms with their loss. Grief counselling is now available to individuals who require help in coming to terms with the death of a loved one. It is vital that grief is successfully overcome in order to enjoy a full and satisfying life afterwards.

Helping Others Cope With Grief

An understanding and compassionate friend can ease the pain of grief by simply listening. The mourner will often recall the life they shared with the deceased and the circumstances of the death. It may be repetitious, so be patient. Allow the outpouring of emotions that frequently accompanies remembering and talking about these events. Simply listening can be difficult, but avoid the tendency to offer advice. The grieving person simply needs a friend to be there, a shoulder to cry on, and not guidance. If it feels appropriate touch and embrace them. Occasionally anger is expressed. Do not take this personally, the mourner is really angry about the loss. Accept this anger as part of normal grieving.

As discussed above the feelings of sadness and loss linger for months. Continue to visit for it is often at this time that the mourner feels most alone. Offer practical help, such as cooking and shopping, if the person is still unwilling to perform these tasks. At certain stages a feeling of despair may engulf the bereaved, as they fear recovery from the loss may never occur. Support and reassurance that these feeling are a normal part of grieving will help them come to terms with the loss. A common suggestion is for the mourner to move from their home as a means of leaving behind past memories. Important decisions like these are best deferred for twelve to eighteen months, when the grief has been resolved. It can be very rewarding to help someone through a period of mourning; this experience can enrich and strengthen the bonds of friendship.

3 EXERCISE

> *Speaking generally, all parts of the body which have a function, if used in moderation and exercised in labours to which each is accustomed, become thereby healthy and well developed, and age slowly; but if left unused and left idle, they become liable to disease, defective in growth, and age quickly.*
>
> Hippocrates

In western society increasing age is associated with a decline in physical activity. The expectation is that after many years of hard work, later life is a time for people to put their feet up and take it easy. While exercise is encouraged in the young and middle-aged, an incorrect assumption that it is unnecessary in later life persists. The community is not used to seeing older people exercising in public; there seems to be a feeling that this is somehow unattractive and improper, and particularly in regards to women. Fortunately recent reports suggest that this trend is changing, with 26 per cent of those over fifty-five years undertaking some form of exercise at least once a week. Of those that engage in exercise, half perform vigorous exercise three times per week.

Many people overestimate the value of their present limited activities, such as a leisurely walk with the dog. Without doubt any activity, no matter how modest, is better than no activity at all. However, to improve fitness and prevent the diseases associated with a sedentary lifestyle, a more active exercise programme needs to be undertaken.

Another false belief which persists is that exercise is excessively risky in later life. The evidence is to the contrary — regular moderate exercise is both beneficial and safe.

Indeed, inactivity causes more problems than exercise, with many physical functions deteriorating with disuse. Lack of exercise is associated with heart disease, high blood pressure, joint stiffness and many other health problems. At least half the decline associated with advancing years is due to inactivity, and not disease or ageing itself. This decline can be prevented and in some cases even reversed by regular activity.

Exercise encourages a more vigorous and active life. This results in more healthy years, living independently and free from chronic ailments. Although to date there is no evidence to suggest that exercise actually prolongs life, there are strong indications that it minimizes dependency and disability while at the same time greatly improving the quality of later life. Research has shown that a 20 per cent improvement in fitness can lead to an extra six to eight years of independence. People are never too old to participate in an appropriate and moderate exercise programme, even those who have been inactive for many years. This chapter will explain the benefits of exercise and how it can be performed safely and effectively.

THE BENEFITS OF EXERCISE

Regular exercise improves many bodily functions. People who exercise can look forward to improved fitness, better general health and move vitality. They report feeling less tired, and have greater stamina to perform their work and recreational activities. Activities which involve physical exertion, such as climbing to a lookout with friends, can be exhilarating events or exhausting trials of endurance. Fit older adults enjoy more of these pleasurable physical activities.

The relationship between exercise and heart function has been extensively studied, with the results indicating that exercise reduces the risk of heart disease. People who lead sedentary lives have twice the death rate from heart ailments than their more active counterparts. This is because exercise improves the efficiency of the heart, lowers blood pressure and produces favourable changes in blood cholesterol levels.

Bones are strengthened and osteoporosis (thinning of the bones) minimized by regular exercise. Muscle tone, strength and flexibility all improve with physical activity. This results in a better posture and fewer back problems. Improved agility also lessens the chance of sustaining serious injuries from an accident or fall. The false impression that exercise leads to a rapid wearing away of the joints is also incorrect, providing there is no pre-existing arthritis. The rhythmic movements of exercise massages the cartilage lining a joint and circulates the fluid within it, thus improving its function. Without regular movement joints become stiff and inflexible, and lose the ability to perform simple movements. When this involves the legs there is an increased risk of falling. The ability to move and remain active strongly influences how long an individual can live independently and maintain a good quality of life.

Many medical conditions can be improved by regular exercise, and sometimes it is even possible to reduce medication. Lower blood pressure and a reduction in blood cholesterol levels are two important benefits from increased physical activity; diabetes is also a common condition in which exercise is a vital part of the treatment. Walking is an excellent way to improve blood circulation to the legs and is therefore beneficial in peripheral vascular disease. In addition, weight loss and maintaining an optimal body weight are more easily achieved when correct eating habits are combined with exercise.

Exercise also improves emotional and psychological health. A more active lifestyle alleviates anxiety and depression. This may be due to the release of chemicals called endorphines which are naturally occurring morphine-like substances produced by the brain. They are released during exercise and their main effects are to relieve pain and elevate mood. This may explain why regular exercise promotes a positive outlook on life, which in turn enables one to cope more easily with personal stress. People who exercise tend to have high self-esteem, and report a general improvement in the quality of their lives.

Many activities can be performed with friends or require belonging to a group that meets regularly. Bowls, golf and tennis are popular sports which involve membership of a club, while walking, jogging and swimming can become enjoyable social activities when undertaken with friends. Besides the physical and emotional benefits of exercise, on a social level it can provide companionship and opportunities to meet new people.

PREPARING FOR EXERCISE

Before starting to exercise it is advisable to undergo a full medical examination. Past and present medical conditions require evaluation, particularly if heart disease, high blood pressure, diabetes, arthritis or excess weight are problems. In all these cases it can be potentially dangerous to embark on an unsupervised exercise programme. For many people this examination is routine and they can start on their chosen activity free of worry. In selected cases the doctor may decide to perform an exercise stress test. This involves measuring the heart's performance when it is subjected to vigorous exercise. Monitors are placed on the chest to record the heart's performance during exercise, which is undertaken on a treadmill or bicycle. The test is stopped if there is excessive fatigue or heart abnormalities develop, and safe limits to exercise are suggested.

A PRESCRIPTION FOR EXERCISE

To minimize the adverse effects of exercise, and at the same time ensure that some benefit is obtained, a FITT exercise programme can be prescribed. This is an abbreviation for the Frequency, Intensity, Time and Type of exercise. These guidelines are for healthy people or those who have had a medical check-up. It will often take many months to reach this level of fitness.

Frequency — three to five times a week.

Intensity — sufficiently vigorous exercise to increase the heart rate.

Time — twenty to thirty minutes (plus warm-up and cool-down periods).

Type — exercise that involves continuous rhythmic movements of large muscle groups, for example walking, jogging,
swimming.

Frequency and Time of Exercise

The individual's fitness before beginning a FITT exercise
programme determines how often and for how long he or she
should exercise. Some people may only manage five minutes
while twenty to thirty minutes is no effort for others. It is
advisable that previously inactive people do not exceed five
to ten minutes per day twice a week in their first weeks of
training. The amount and frequency of physical activity can
be slowly increased, and it may take three to six months to
achieve an adequate level of fitness. Too rapid an increase
can be dangerous — 'Start low, go slow' encapsulates this
approach to exercise.

The final goal of this programme is to be exercising for
twenty to thirty minutes three to five times each week. More frequent exercising can result in injuries, while activities performed only once or twice each week will not sustain an
adequate level of fitness. Exercising on alternate days allows
for a period of rest between activities.

Intensity of Exercise

Aerobic exercises involve delivering more oxygen to the
active muscles. The heart and lungs must therefore work
harder and more efficiently, causing the heart and breathing
rate to rise. A certain amount of stress is necessary for aerobic
fitness to develop, but this must be carefully balanced against
the hazards of exceeding safe limits of activity. It is therefore
important to monitor the intensity of the exercises performed.
To establish a 'safety limit' it is necessary to measure the *heart
rate*, to ask a person how she or he *feels*, and to perform a
'*talk test*'.

The term 'target exercise heart rate' is used to describe the
rate at which the heart must be pumping to improve fitness,
while remaining within the 'safety limit'. It is calculated as
follows:

1. Measure the *resting heart rate* (usually seventy to eighty beats per minute).

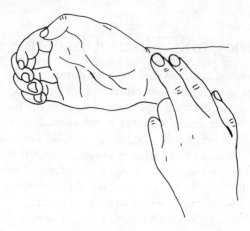

FIGURE 3.1 Measuring the heart rate.

The pulse can be felt by placing the index and middle fingers on the wrist just below the base of the thumb. Count the number of pulse beats in fifteen seconds and multiply it by four to calculate beats per minute.

2. Calculate the *maximum heart rate*.
   During exercise the heart rate increases until exhaustion occurs. This point is the *maximum heart rate*. It decreases with advancing years and is calculated by subtracting a person's age from 220.

$$\text{maximum heart rate} = 220 - \text{age}$$

3. Consider the individual's level of fitness.
   The difference between *resting heart rate* and *maximum heart rate* is the *heart rate reserve*. The rate at which to exercise varies between 60 and 80 per cent of the heart rate reserve according to fitness.

Unfit   — 60 per cent of heart rate reserve
Average fitness — 70 to 75 per cent of heart rate reserve
Fit   — 80 per cent of heart rate reserve

4. Calculate the *target exercise heart rate.*

$$\begin{array}{c}\text{target}\\\text{exercise}\\\text{heart rate}\end{array} = \left[\begin{array}{c}\text{maximum}\\\text{heart rate}\end{array} - \begin{array}{c}\text{resting}\\\text{heart}\\\text{rate}\end{array}\right] \times \frac{60 \text{ to } 80}{100} + \begin{array}{c}\text{resting}\\\text{heart}\\\text{rate}\end{array}$$

Example A: Fit person aged sixty years
1. Resting pulse 70 beats per minute.
2. Maximum pulse rate = 220 − 70 = 150.
3. Fit, therefore exercise at 80 per cent of heart rate reserve.

Apply the formula:

$$\begin{array}{c}\text{target}\\\text{exercise}\\\text{heart rate}\end{array} = \left[\begin{array}{c}\text{maximum}\\\text{heart rate}\end{array} - \begin{array}{c}\text{resting}\\\text{heart}\\\text{rate}\end{array}\right] \times \frac{60 \text{ to } 80}{100} + \begin{array}{c}\text{resting}\\\text{heart}\\\text{rate}\end{array}$$

$$= (150 - 70) \times \frac{80}{100} + 70$$

$$= 134 \text{ beats per minute}$$

Example B: Unfit person aged sixty years
1. Resting pulse 80 beats per minute.
2. Maximum pulse rate = 220 − 80 = 140.
3. Unfit, therefore exercise at 60 per cent of heart rate reserve.
   Apply the formula:

$$\begin{array}{c}\text{target}\\\text{exercise}\\\text{heart rate}\end{array} = \left[\begin{array}{c}\text{maximum}\\\text{heart rate}\end{array} - \begin{array}{c}\text{resting}\\\text{heart}\\\text{rate}\end{array}\right] \times \frac{60 \text{ to } 80}{100} + \begin{array}{c}\text{resting}\\\text{heart}\\\text{rate}\end{array}$$

$$= (140 - 80) \times \frac{60}{100} + 80$$

$$= 116 \text{ beats per minute}$$

As fitness improves it is sometimes safer for an older person to maintain their pulse rate at the same level (e.g. 60 per cent of heart rate reserve) and exercise for a longer period of time. An exercise stress test is another accurate way of monitoring the heart's response to exercise, and to determine safe limits. This is particularly important at higher levels of exertion or if heart disease is present. Heart rate should not be used as the only measure of performance.

A reliable and more convenient method of assessing the correct intensity of exercise is simply to be guided by how a person feels. To obtain any benefit from exercise a person should be performing moderately hard work, but also be feeling comfortable and not over stressed. While exercising it is acceptable to be mildly breathless, but a person should still be able to carry on a conversation. This is called the 'talk test'. If a person is unable to talk comfortably, then the limits of safety have been exceeded. Pain is another obvious indication of excessive exertion. It is the body's means of conveying that there is a problem which must not be ignored. After exercise most people should feel pleasantly tired but not exhausted or strained.

Types of Exercise

A balanced activity programme incorporates the three basic types of exercise — aerobic, mobility and strengthening. They are interrelated, for example a person who is strong and supple is more easily able to improve his or her aerobic fitness.

Aerobic Exercise

Stamina is improved by aerobic exercise. It involves an increase in the work performed by the heart and lungs, whose function it is to maintain an adequate supply of blood to the exercising muscles. As a result the heart functions more efficiently and the body's endurance increases. This form of exercise lowers the risk of heart attack, reduces blood pressure, facilitates weight loss and improves fitness. Aerobic exercise should involve the continuous rhythmical use of large muscle groups, particularly the legs. There are a wide range of aerobic activities and choice is largely determined by an individual's level of fitness. Most older people should start with a less strenuous exercise such as walking. As fitness improves, they can progress to more vigorous exercises, for example brisk walking, jogging or cycling. Similar commonsense advice applies to dancing and swimming, which are also aerobic activities.

Mobility Exercises

Joints tend to stiffen if they are not used. Mobility exercises improve the range of joint movements, stretching muscles and ligaments which become more supple and mobile. The overall result is increased flexibility, agility of movement and improved posture. Stretching exercises should be performed in a warm environment and after a gentle warm-up. It is advisable to do them slowly and without 'bouncing'. After completing mobility exercises the muscles should feel pleasantly stretched, but not painful or strained. Many people find that gentle mobility exercises improve the movement in arthritic joints.

Strengthening Exercises

Improved strength enables a person to remain mobile, self-reliant and active. If unexpected physical demands are confronted, this extra reserve enables the body to cope better and reduces the risk of injury. Muscle size and strength also affect appearance and posture. Many exercises strengthen muscles, however training with heavy weights should be avoided, as it can cause a dangerous rise in blood pressure.

Planning an Exercise Programme

Warm-up and cool-down periods are an essential part of a safe exercise programme. They should be performed for five to ten minutes at the beginning and end of the session. Low intensity exercises (e.g. slow walking or swimming) together with stretching movements form their basis. Warm-up activities prepare the heart and lungs for the increased demands of exertion. In addition they improve flexibility and strength which prevents damage to joints and muscles. The cool-down period allows the heart to slowly settle back to normal. Too rapid a reduction can result in dangerous irregular heart beats as the heart continues to beat rapidly while insufficient blood is returning to it from the now resting body. Slowly cooling down also prevents muscle stiffness and soreness, and it promotes a sense of relaxed wellbeing.

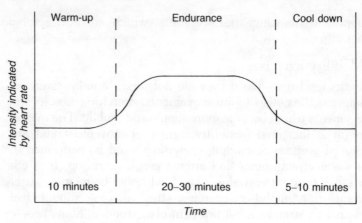

FIGURE 3.2 A typical exercise session.

As discussed earlier, an exercise programme should start slowly, well within safe levels of activity, and increase very gradually as fitness improves. For an older person less intense exercise performed for a longer time is preferable to short periods of over-exertion. Moderation and being attentive to the body's response to exercise will help ensure a beneficial and safe exercise programme. Finally, a person who has been inactive for some time should not be deterred from starting — any exercise is better than none. There is no set level of exertion that must be achieved before some benefits are felt.

Choosing an Exercise Programme

Personal needs and preferences play an important part in determining the type of activity undertaken. Some people prefer group or club sports while others choose to exercise by themselves. When selecting an activity it is important to keep in mind that it should be enjoyable and easily incorporated into the daily routine. Once an exercise becomes unpleasant or a chore it is usually not long before it is stopped. Such considerations as proximity to home, travelling involved and cost and equipment require careful consideration in the planning stages if the activity is to be successfully continued for many years.

After retirement financial considerations are particularly important, as many people then have a fixed income.

Traditional sports such as bowls, table tennis, tennis and golf are inexpensive, while walking involves no cost apart from a good pair of shoes. Fitness trails in local parks are available for use by people of all ages, however care must be taken that a person is sufficiently fit to perform all the exercises. An increasing number of local councils are organizing activities specifically designed for older adults. These include aqua-aerobics and swimming in the local pool, aerobic classes and walking clubs. Contacting a council's activities officer or the regional community centre is the easiest way to find out what is available. In addition to these activities playing a ball game or flying a kite with grandchildren provides both enjoyable and invigorating exercise. Choosing active hobbies is another inexpensive way to exercise. Gardening, fishing, redecorating, woodwork and bush walking offer varying levels of pleasant exertion.

A further consideration is the amount of energy required to exercise. It is stating the obvious to suggest that different exercises involve varying degrees of exertion. For example walking is a less vigorous activity than jogging. The unit that measures the amount of energy used or METabolized is the MET. One MET is the amount of energy the body requires at rest. Listed below are different activities and the amount of energy (METS) each requires.

In addition to becoming involved in specific sporting or recreational activities, exercise can easily be incorporated into the daily routine. The many labour saving devices of modern society encourage a sedentary lifestyle. Walking rather than driving, washing the car, working around the house and using stairs instead of lifts are everyday activities which contribute to improved fitness.

There are a wide variety of sports and activities available to the older person who wishes to improve his or her fitness. There is evidence to suggest that a combination of different sports may be preferable, since each can be beneficial in different ways. For example playing bowls on some days and brisk walking on others combines the social advantages of a group sport with the aerobic fitness of walking. Below are some of the more popular choices, with explanations of what each has to offer.

TABLE 3.1 Energy used (METabolized) for various activities
(National Heart Foundation of Australia)

Activity	METs used
resting	1
writing, sewing, dressing, driving	1–2
sweeping, lawn bowling, fishing	2–3
walking (4 km/h)	
housework — bed making, hanging clothes, vacuuming	3–4
gardening,	
10 pin bowling	
walking (5 km/h)	
golf (pulling cart)	
table tennis	
sailing	
scrubbing floors	4–5
lawn mowing, digging	
sex	
tennis (doubles)	
dancing	
swimming (slow)	
tennis (singles)	5–6
swimming	
walking (6 km/h)	6–7
skiing (water and snow)	
jogging (8 km/h)	7–8
gymnastics	
basketball	

Lawn bowls

Lawn bowls is one of the most popular sports in Australia. It improves joint flexibility and requires good co-ordination. Participants belong to clubs, so there is plenty of opportunity to develop new friendships. The level of social involvement varies according to the individual. Some people enjoy the administrative running of the club and become involved in committees that organize the club's activities, while others may prefer a lower profile, enjoying the companionship and pleasure of a game once every week or so.

Bowls is not a sport that greatly improves fitness and is best combined with an aerobic activity.

Golf

Golf is another sport which improves skill rather than fitness. Although it involves a lot of walking, the 'stop-start' nature of the game does not allow the heart rate to reach aerobic levels. The level of fitness achieved is higher if the golfer wheels her or his clubs in a buggy, rather than driving a golf cart. The strength and flexibility of the back and shoulders in particular improve with golf. In order to increase heart and lung fitness it is advisable to participate in an aerobic sport on the days that golf is not played. Like those who play bowls, golfers often belong to a club, which encourages social contact and friendships.

Swimming

Swimming in a heated pool is balanced aerobic exercise. It has the advantage of providing buoyancy and support for the body in water. This is particularly important for the overweight or those with joint problems which may be aggravated by the jarring of weight-bearing exercises such as jogging. For people with back pains swimming is an excellent form of exercise as it strengthens the back muscles and improves flexibility without the risk of injury. In practice few people are sufficiently expert to swim at a rate fast enough to produce aerobic levels of fitness.

Water aerobics is a recent adaptation, combining aerobics with the advantages of swimming. This group activity is beneficial for those with joint and back problems without requiring the ability to swim. The warmth is soothing and relaxing, while the water protects the joints from the force of gravity and offers resistance for the muscles to work against. As with other group activities it provides an opportunity to socialize.

Dancing

Dancing ranges from formal ballroom dancing to the more contemporary aerobic dancing, with many forms in between (e.g. square dancing, ethnic dancing). It is primarily a recreational activity which has only recently been recognized as a form of aerobic exercise. Individual variations are catered for by changing the complexity and intensity of the dance. Care must be taken to choose a dance class which suits an individual's present level of fitness, as vigorous dancing can be equivalent to playing competitive sport. Dancing provides the opportunity to meet new people and develop friendships. It offers the social benefits of an enjoyable group activity, in addition to improving stamina, co-ordination and flexibility.

Tennis

Tennis is an excellent sport that is often started in youth and continued throughout life. However, people contemplating playing tennis for the first time in later life or after a long absence from sporting activities, should begin by first increasing their aerobic fitness. Only after attaining a good level of physical fitness is it safe to participate in tennis and other 'faster' sports.

While a game of singles is an excellent aerobic exercise, a doubles match is less energetic but offers the opportunity to meet and exercise with friends. The popularity of this sport has led to the establishment of Veteran's Tennis, where people of varying fitness and skill can play at their local clubs, or compete internationally in competitions specifically organized for the mature-aged player.

Exercise Classes

Attending exercise classes is an ideal way for unfit people to increase their level of activity. The instructor demonstrates the exercises to the class, and makes sure that participants perform them correctly. Often the exercises are performed to music and include warm-up and cool-down periods as well as stretching and endurance exercises. There are generally different classes for people of differing fitness. For the inexperienced, it is important to start at an introductory level specifically designed for older adults, and graduate to more strenuous exercises as fitness improves. Exercise classes are both a safe and enjoyable way to exercise. They are available through private gyms and increasingly from local community recreation centres.

Walking

Human beings were made to walk. Walking is a convenient, inexpensive, safe and effective exercise that can be undertaken by any person, at any time and in any place. Walking is particularly suitable for people who have been inactive or prefer a less vigorous form of exercise. With improved fitness the time spent exercising or the distance walked can be increased. This is preferable to increasing the intensity of exercise — longer periods of moderate activity (e.g. walking) produce similar benefits to short periods of more vigorous forms of exercising (e.g. jogging). Walking is also safer for older people starting an exercise programme.

Brisk walking provides all the benefits of aerobic exercise without the risk of injury associated with other energetic activities. No special equipment is necessary apart from a good pair of walking or jogging shoes. This brisk form of walking is also termed aerobic or power walking. It involves taking long purposeful strides while swinging the arms to shoulder height.

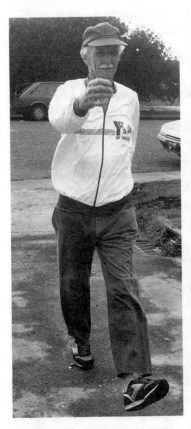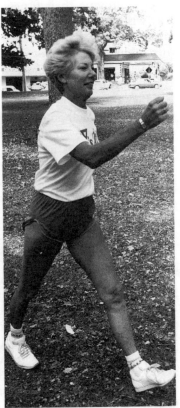

FIGURE 3.3 Aerobic walking.

Warm-up exercises should be performed before walking. Walk at a comfortable pace, working a little bit harder than normal so that there is a feeling of being slightly out of breath. The pace should not be so fast as to result in excessive breathlessness and it should still be possible to carry on a conversation (talk test). Avoid walking up steep hills and against the wind, particularly when first starting a fitness programme, as this can significantly increase the work of exercise. Walking can also be a relaxing and social activity to be enjoyed in the company of friends or by walking in parks and the bush.

Jogging

After improving their fitness by brisk walking, some people may wish to try jogging. It is most important not to do too much too soon. Pain and excessive tiredness are warning signs that should not be ignored — either slow down or stop exercising. As a rough guide, if an individual can walk five kilometres (three miles) in forty-five minutes, then he or she is sufficiently fit to start slow jogging. It is best to begin by interspersing small amounts of slow running with the already established brisk walking, repeating this cycle for up to twenty minutes. As fitness improves the proportion of jogging can be slowly increased by one to two minutes each week, but never more than 10 per cent on the previous week's running. Jogging allows a person to achieve a high level of fitness.

THE HAZARDS OF EXERCISE

A common excuse for not exercising is the fear of injuring a body unused to such activity. It is worth remembering, however, that the risk of death is greater from driving a car than from exercise. There is a definite but small risk of suffering a heart attack while exercising, but people who do have underlying heart disease. There is no evidence that increased activity causes problems if the heart is healthy. Heart disease is partly due to a lack of exercise, together with other risk factors such as smoking, high cholesterol and being overweight. People who exercise regularly throughout their lives are less likely to suffer a heart attack than those who are sedentary. In fact, inactivity is a greater risk to the health of an older person than sensible moderate exercise.

Injuries to muscles, ligaments and joints are more common in people who exercise infrequently. Sore muscles, sprains and painful joints are usually a reflection of inadequate preparation or excessively intense and prolonged activity. Studies have shown that the risk of injury increases if a person exercises more than three times each week, or for longer than one hour. Although the damage is usually minor, if it is ignored more serious problems can develop. These risks can be minimized by proper planning, correct equipment and gradually increasing the amount of exertion as fitness improves.

Overcoming the Hazards

Much of what follows could be termed commonsense advice; injuries are preventable so it is important to consider ways of ensuring that exercise remains safe. Preparing the correct equipment is essential. For walking and jogging specially designed impact absorbent shoes should be worn. These cushion the trauma suffered when the foot strikes the ground and this protects the joints of the lower limbs and back. Loose, comfortable and light-weight clothing is most appropriate for aerobic exercises, because overheating can occur. Similarly extreme environmental conditions are best avoided, for example in summer exercise during the coolest time of the day. To prevent dehydration make sure that fluids lost in perspiration are replaced by drinking before and after exertion. Exercise should be avoided after eating a meal (wait two hours) or drinking alcohol and during periods of ill health.

Gentle warm-up and stretching exercises before starting, and a cool-down period at the end of a work-out are necessary if sporting injuries are to be avoided. These should be performed even in preparation for walking or playing a social game of tennis. It is wrong to assume that only professional athletes need to perform warm-up and cooling down exercises.

Many problems are related to extremes in exercising. A moderate exercise programme performed on alternate days is ideal. Start slowly and gradually increase the amount of activity over a period of weeks or months. Lengthening the time spent performing moderate exercise will improve fitness and is less likely to cause injuries. It is advisable to delay playing competitive sports until an adequate level of fitness has been achieved; the amount of exertion cannot be safely predicted or monitored during competition, and this increases the risk of injury.

Discomfort or pain is the body's way of signalling that a problem has developed, commonly in a joint, muscle or ligament. Stop exercising if an injury is sustained. Faintness, dizziness, nausea, undue fatigue or feeling light-headed and sweaty are indications that the exercise is too stressful. Chest pain, significant breathlessness and swollen ankles are other warning signs. In these circumstances, especially if chest pain develops during exertion, it is important to consult a doctor as heart disease may be the cause.

As discussed earlier a full medical check-up is advisable before embarking on an exercise programme, particularly if a person has not exercised for some time or suffers from health problems. Arthritis, high blood pressure, heart disease, diabetes and obesity are common ailments that require assessment prior to exercising. Modifications can be made to an exercise programme so that all the activities can be performed safely. During an illness exercise should be stopped, and after recovering started again at a lower level. It can then be gradually increased until the previous fitness level has been reached.

MOTIVATION

Many older adults are reluctant to change their present comfortable but sedentary lifestyle. For this reason extra motivation and incentives may be required. The following suggestions should prove helpful in starting, and continuing, exercise on a regular basis:

- exercise with a friend or in a group;
- join a club, for example, a bowling, tennis or walking club;
- choose an exercise which suits personal interests and lifestyle;
- set realistic short and long term goals;

- record improvements;
- reward achievements;
- plan activities in advance;
- incorporate exercise into the daily routine;
- introduce variety, for example combine bowling and walking, or vary the walking route;
- remember that exercise can be a means of relaxing.

For exercise to become an integral part of life it should be enjoyable and adapted to personal needs and interests. The final responsibility rests with the individual, who will reap the significant rewards that increased activity can bring.

4 FOOD AND NUTRITION

'You are what you eat.'

A balanced diet is fundamental to good health. Poor nutrition predisposes to the development of certain diseases. Scurvy, for instance, was once common, and results from a vitamin C deficiency. Although some nutritional problems in older people may not present as obvious symptoms of an illness, they may have a major influence on health and wellbeing. Poor nutrition can cause physical and mental deterioration in any person, and in the case of an older person this is often incorrectly attributed to ageing.

Research confirms that 60 per cent of deaths in Australia are from diseases associated with diet, particularly heart disease and cancer. In addition, food plays a significant role in diabetes, obesity and tooth decay. Many people in modern western societies die from simply over-eating the wrong foods.

Healthy eating is not a matter of denial or hardship, but should be approached as the learning of new and improved eating habits. The emphasis is on moderation rather than restriction. Life must remain enjoyable, food palatable, and the suggested changes permanent. Although modifications may be significant, they should not be so drastic as to prevent their continuation, or so unusual as to limit social activities which involve eating.

Eating should be interesting and enjoyable. This is best achieved by taking in a variety of foods, which also helps ensure that deficiencies do not develop. The emphasis should be on the quality, not the quantity, of food eaten. Moderation is also an important consideration — too much or too little of any food can result in an unbalanced diet. It is important to include foods containing fibre, for example, yet excess fibre may result in deficiencies of zinc and iron. A balanced, sensible approach to food should also allow the occasional 'fun foods', which are enjoyable to eat but not necessarily nutritious. Of the twenty-one meals eaten each week, the occasional indiscretion will do no harm provided the other meals are healthy. Professor Sali summarizes this in *The One Page Good Diet Book*: 'What matters most is what you *usually* eat, not what you *occasionally* eat'.

Food serves many functions in addition to supplying the energy for living. Eating should be enjoyable and mealtimes occasions to relax. Food is often the focus of family, communal and other social activities, when people arrange to meet and eat together. Religious events are also sometimes celebrated with special foods. It is necessary to consider these social factors when planning a healthy diet.

In Australia poor nutrition can be attributed to dietary habits, and in most circumstances not the availability of food. There is a tremendous variety of foods from which to choose. Generally fresh produce should be purchased, since it is more nutritious and less expensive than processed foods. Advertising influences our choices and unfortunately the packaged and processed foods are those most widely promoted. This combined with the conveniences of modern society, especially the motor car, leads many people to eat more than their body requires. Gradually, however, people are responding to the increased amount of information available on healthy eating, and those who have adopted new eating patterns often comment that they feel better, and have more energy to enjoy an active life. The aim of this chapter is to provide up-to-date information on current trends in nutrition. It is never too late to adopt new eating habits, and doing so will result in greater vitality, less illness and a better quality of life.

NUTRITION AND LATER LIFE
Longevity

Food and nutrition are recognized as having some influence on how long we will live. Restricting the intake of food has been shown to prolong the lives of laboratory animals, yet this apparent extension of life may in fact be the animal living to its full life expectancy, with over-eating in the 'normal' animals resulting in the premature development of diseases which shorten their lives. It has been suggested that the extra amount of food eaten results in more chemical reactions in cells, and the production of additional free radicals that cause ageing and disease. This remains to be verified, however.

Although these are interesting ideas, it can be misleading to extend the findings of animal experiments and apply them to humans. For example, malnutrition is the likely outcome if a person's food intake is significantly reduced, and based on the present information food restriction cannot be recommended as a safe method of extending life. It is also unlikely ever to be proven that food restriction prolongs life in human beings — few are willing to subject themselves to a lifetime of such hardship and deprivation. Indeed, there are some people who suggest the opposite is true, and that those who are slightly overweight are likely to live longer. However, these suggestions have been dismissed as being biased by smokers who have a higher incidence of disease but are less likely to be overweight. The present recommendation for a long and healthy life is for a person to eat a balanced diet and maintain an ideal weight throughout life.

Nutritional Problems

Ageing causes a number of normal changes in the body that should be taken into account when considering nutrition. There is a decrease in the body's metabolism, for example, which when combined with the sedentary lifestyle frequently associated with later life, reduces the body's energy (kilojoule) requirements. Those who eat the same amount of food will therefore become overweight. Importantly, there is no reduction in the amount of nutrients such as protein, vitamins and minerals the body requires, so if insufficient food is eaten malnutrition can occur. Those in later life are therefore caught between obesity if the food intake is not modified, and inadequate nutrition if it is excessively reduced. The ideal is to eat highly nutritious food while ensuring that the total energy intake is decreased.

In practice this means eating fewer processed and fatty foods; these are high in kilojoules and contain fewer nutrients than wholesome foods such as fruit, vegetables and wholegrain cereals. Exercise is also a vital factor, allowing a person to eat more food (ensuring an adequate intake of nutrients) without gaining weight. As we saw in the previous chapter, it is advisable that people of *all* ages exercise regularly, and it is possible to do so safely in later life.

Appetite may be affected by the decrease in taste and smell that frequently occurs in later life. Less saliva makes chewing more difficult and changes in the amount of digestive juices also affect the absorption of nutrients from food. It is also very important to care for teeth if a balanced diet is to be eaten, since fibrous foods, a necessary part of the diet, are difficult to eat without natural teeth. For too long dentists have enthusiastically removed the few remaining teeth of older people, so that dentures can be more easily fitted. Fortunately, this attitude is now changing.

A number of diseases can affect nutrition, causing problems that range from difficulties with buying and preparing food, to prescribed drugs interfering with the body's normal functions. Arthritis and stroke, for instance, can limit a person's ability to shop for and purchase food, as well as make preparation and cooking more difficult. Some supermarkets accept phone orders and also offer home delivery for people who cannot shop themselves. Drugs such as antihistamines and antidepressants may stimulate the appetite, leading to obesity. Many people take fluid tablets which increase the body's potassium requirements while cholestyramine, a powder commonly used to lower cholesterol, reduces the absorption of important vitamins. Tablets to relieve pain, often taken for arthritis, may affect the bowel, causing indigestion and constipation. Unfortunately it is often the people taking these medications who can least tolerate such problems. It is therefore advisable to limit the number of medications to those that are absolutely necessary and to take them in the lowest effective dose. More generally, many illnesses depress the appetite, leading to a vicious circle of poor nutrition with slower healing and a prolonged period of recovery.

As mentioned, social involvement has an impact on eating. Meals are often a time for meeting with other people. Those who live alone often do not make the effort to prepare and cook meals for themselves. This is particularly true of widowers, who may also not be very experienced in cooking. It is not uncommon for soup, toast and tea to be eaten instead of proper meals by people who live alone and find meal preparation too much trouble.

Involvement in social activities and clubs can provide the opportunity to discuss recipes and cooking methods. It may also provide enjoyable interaction for otherwise lonely people, who are at greatest risk of malnutrition. Their appetite may be poor, and they may rely on processed foods which require no preparation, but which have little nutritional value. Bereavement and depression usually affect appetite and it is particularly important during these times to ensure that the food eaten is highly nutritious.

There is a wide variation in the social circumstances of older people. Although most remain in their own homes and cook for themselves, some choose to live with their families or in communal accommodation. Problems in the latter situation, particularly, can arise because the individual has little or no control over the types of food provided. Migrants, who are used to eating traditional foods, may find such situations especially difficult. In addition, care must be taken to ensure that when food is cooked in bulk not too many of the nutrients are lost. Fortunately many establishments now consult with dieticians when planning their menus.

A frequent complaint is that it is difficult to purchase the smaller quantities of food that an older couple or single person requires. Self-serve shopping or buying larger quantities to be shared with friends are possible solutions here. Frozen vegetables retain most of their nutrients, and are able to be used in small quantities without wasting the remainder. Because frozen vegetables are pre-cut, people with arthritis may find them particularly convenient. Cooking extra quantities that can be frozen and eaten on another occasion also helps those who find cooking a chore, while cold meals with salad, meat or fish, bread and fruit, are both simple and nutritious. Finally, those who cannot cook for themselves due to ill health can obtain a cooked meal from 'meals on wheels'.

COMMON HEALTH PROBLEMS AND DIET

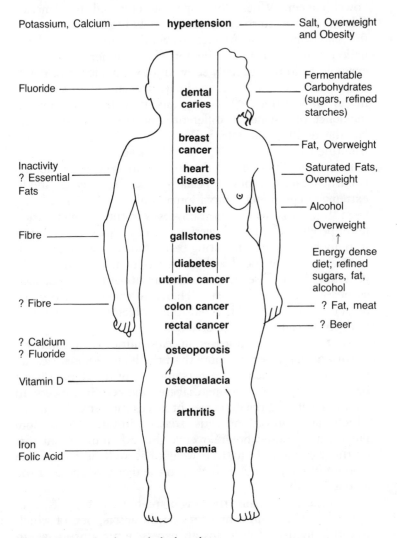

Nutritional deficiency

Nutritional excess

Potassium, Calcium ———— **hypertension** ———— Salt, Overweight and Obesity

Fluoride ———————— **dental caries** ———— Fermentable Carbohydrates (sugars, refined starches)

breast cancer

Inactivity ? Essential Fats ———— **heart disease** ———— Fat, Overweight

Saturated Fats, Overweight

liver —— Alcohol

Fibre ———————— **gallstones** —— Overweight ↑ Energy dense diet; refined sugars, fat, alcohol

diabetes

uterine cancer

? Fibre ———————— **colon cancer** —— ? Fat, meat

rectal cancer —— ? Beer

? Calcium ? Fluoride ———————— **osteoporosis**

Vitamin D ———————— **osteomalacia**

arthritis

Iron Folic Acid ———————— **anaemia**

FIGURE 4.1 Conditions linked to diet.

A balanced diet is essential for the maintenance of good health, and, as noted, poor nutrition is associated with the development of a number of diseases. Population studies have revealed that the incidence of disease varies in different countries. For example, the incidence of stomach cancer is high amongst the Japanese, while Americans suffer from more bowel cancer. When the Japanese migrated to America (Hawaii) this pattern changed, and they began to suffer from the same diseases as Americans. Similar studies have been undertaken in Australia. Migrants from southern Europe, for example, who traditionally showed a low incidence of bowel cancer and heart disease, gradually succumbed to these ill-nesses in Australia. This suggests that the variation in incidence of diseases in different countries is not inherited, but the result of lifestyle, with diet being a significant con-tributing factor.

It is generally accepted that poor nutrition in developing countries leads to illness, especially infectious diseases, and in extreme circumstances starvation and ultimately death. It has been shown that as nutrition improves in these communities, fewer people suffer from infections and they live longer. After initially benefiting from eating better foods, however, a point is reached where the death rate starts to rise again. This is generally due to diseases prevalent in affluent societies, such as heart disease and cancer. Therefore there is an optimal level of nutrition, which avoids the problems associated with both insufficient and excessive food intake.

Most diet-related diseases in Australia arise from over-nutrition, that is, eating more than the body requires. *Obesity* is common and increases a person's risk of developing heart disease, high blood pressure, diabetes and certain cancers. In addition, carrying the extra weight places more stress on joints which can aggravate arthritis. *Diabetes* in later life is more prevalent in those who are overweight and an important part of the treatment is to lose weight, as well as reduce the amount of fat, sugar and alcohol in the diet, and increase the amount of fibre.

Heart disease remains the single greatest cause of death in Australia. There are a number of risk factors, one of which is eating food that contains an excessive amount of fat, in particular saturated fat and cholesterol. Fish, fruit and vegetables, on the other hand, are believed to have a beneficial effect in preventing heart disease. It is advisable to eat more of these foods and reduce the total amount of fat in the diet. Polyunsaturated or monounsaturated oils can be used when fat is required. The recent moderate reduction in heart disease has been partly attributed to healthier eating and better control of blood pressure.

High blood pressure can be lowered in some people by reducing their intake of salt. In addition potassium, present in fruit and wholegrain cereals, is believed to prevent high blood pressure by helping the body get rid of excess salt. Calcium and dietary fibre are also factors that favourably affect blood pressure, while excess alcohol causes it to rise.

Not surprisingly, diseases of the digestive tract are also often caused by what we eat. *Diverticulitis*, (inflamed pouches in the bowel wall), *irritable colon* (spasms in the bowel), *constipation* and *haemorrhoids* are all associated with inadequate fibre intake. *Gall stones*, which are often composed of cholesterol, are more prevalent in people who are overweight and who eat too many sugars.

There has been much interest and speculation on the relationship between diet and *cancer*. It has been postulated that 35 per cent of cancers are related to diet, slightly more than due to smoking (30 per cent). *Bowel cancer* is reduced in people who consume cruciferous vegetables (cauliflower, broccoli, cabbage, brussel sprouts). Dietary fibre also protects against this cancer because it absorbs water, diluting possible cancer-causing agents. Fibre also moves food through the body more quickly, reducing the time these substances are exposed to the bowel. Smoked or salt-cured foods such as smoked fish and corned beef are also associated with bowel cancer; they contain nitrites which are converted to cancer inducing agents. Vitamin C stops this conversion and so reduces the risk of cancer. A high fat diet also increases the risk of bowel cancer. It is suggested that the release of extra bile to digest the fat promotes the production of cancer-causing substances. Alcohol is associated with cancer of the throat and bowel, especially in smokers. The relationship between these cancers and diet and alcohol is not difficult to accept, because there is direct contact between the affected organ and the agent believed to be causing the cancer.

In women the connection between *cancer of the breast and womb* and diet is not as clear, but studies have revealed that those who are overweight and eat too much fat are more likely to develop these cancers. Fat and cholesterol are used in the formation of the sex hormones. The excess fat may lead to the production of extra hormones which in turn act on the breast and womb which are sensitive to them. It is possible then, that dietary imbalances are associated with these problems, which can therefore be rectified.

There are a number of vitamins and minerals that act as antioxidants. The free radical theory of ageing and disease (see p. 12) suggests that dangerous free radicals are produced in the body as the result of oxidation. These antioxidants 'mop up' the free radicals before they can damage important structures in the cells. Zinc, copper, selenium and vitamins A, C, and E are all antioxidants which early research indicates may lower the incidence of some cancers. Beta-carotine, which the body can convert to vitamin A, has been demonstrated to reduce the risk of lung, bowel and skin cancer. It is present in yellow-orange fruit and vegetables (carrots, pumkin, apricots, pawpaw), and green vegetables (broccoli, spinach). A number of the other vitamins and minerals have been shown to protect against cancer in animals, but more research needs to be done to determine if these benefits apply to humans. The present information indicates that it is sensible to eat foods such as fruit and vegetables that contain these valuable antioxidants. There is no evidence to suggest that greater protection can be achieved by taking larger doses of antioxidants in tablet form.

Osteoporosis can be prevented by taking in an adequate amount of calcium. Dairy products are also recommended as protective against cancer.

Examining the types of food that cause disease reveals a common pattern. A diet which is high in kilojoules, fat and sugar but low in fibre is associated with diseases which are prevalent in affluent societies, such as heart disease and cancer. Many preventive properties are present in foods such as wholegrain cereals, fruit and vegetables, and these should be eaten as part of a healthy diet.

THE NUTRIENTS IN FOOD

The vital nutrients in food are carbohydrates, protein, fat, vitamins, minerals and water. They provide the energy for living and the materials necessary for the maintenance and repair of vital organs. People require the same nutrients in later life as in their younger years. Reduced activity and slowing of the metabolism with age means fewer kilojoules and therefore less food is required. If all nutrients are to be present but the meals smaller, there must be careful consideration of the quality and types of food eaten.

The current recommendations for the sources of energy (kilojoules) from the different nutrients are: carbohydrates 50 per cent; fat 30 per cent; protein 12–14 per cent.

Carbohydrates

Carbohydrates form the basis of a balanced diet and provide most of the 'fuel' for living. The main foods in the category are cereals, fruits, vegetables, legumes (lentils, baked beans, chickpeas) and sugars. They are also an important source of vitamins. Thiamin is present in cereals, while fruit and vegetables contain vitamin C and beta-carotene (vitamin A). These foods are low in fat and should be substituted for those containing high amounts of fat. Carbohydrates are made up of three components: sugars (refined carbohydrates); starches (unrefined carbohydrates), and fibre.

Simple sugars are very sweet and should only be eaten in small quantities. They include glucose, cane or 'normal' sugar (sucrose), fruit sugar (fructose) and milk sugar (lactose). Unrefined sugars are commonly found in cereal crops such as wheat, oats, rice and corn. From these raw ingredients bread, breakfast cereals and pasta are made. When eaten, these foods are slowly absorbed, causing a modest but sustained rise in blood glucose levels. Hunger is therefore satisfied for a longer period of time. This is also why starches are important in preventing obesity and controlling diabetes. Following is a list of ways to reduce the intake of refined carbohydrates and increase unrefined carbohydrates in the diet.

Suggestions for reducing refined carbohydrates in the diet
- Limit soft drinks; substitute unsweetened fruit juices (no more than one to two glasses per day) or water;
- Avoid adding sugar to foods, for example tea, coffee, cereals and fruit, and choose foods with the least sugar (check the labels). Allow no more than three to six teaspoons of sugar per day;
- Substitute fruit, cereals and wholemeal bread for desserts and snacks.

Suggestions for increasing unrefined carbohydrates
- Substitute wholemeal and wholegrain foods for those that are refined, for example, brown or wholemeal bread, wholemeal pasta, brown rice, rolled oats instead of white bread, pasta, white rice, refined cereals (rice bubbles, cornflakes);
- Include vegetables, preferably fresh, in meals;
- Prepare salads as a side dish;
- Increase the portions of vegetables and eat smaller amounts of red and white meats;
- Replace some meat meals with legumes, that is, lentils, dried peas and beans;
- Serve fresh fruit with most meals.

Fibre

The interest in fibre began in the 1960s when Dr Denis Burkett noted the absence of many 'western' diseases in tribal Africans. He suggested that this was the result of their different lifestyle, in particular the significantly higher intake of dietary fibre. Despite modifications and refinement of this original idea, the basic recommendation to increase the amount of fibre in the diet remains. High fibre foods include wholemeal bread, wholegrain cereals, fruit, vegetables and nuts. Food from animals, for example meat and milk, is low in fibre.

The main source of fibre is plant food. Fibre is not digested in the small bowel, where the absorption of most nutrients occurs, but passes as 'roughage' into the large bowel. There a small proportion of the fibre is broken down by bacteria. The remainder continues through the bowel to be expelled as waste. Although fibre is not a nutrient, the old idea of it being a single inactive substance, simply passing unchanged through the digestive system, has been challenged by new findings.

There are two main types of fibre, soluble and insoluble. Within these groups there are a number of substances, each with different properties. Unprocessed bran — the husks of wheat — was the first to capture public attention. This and other cereals contain insoluble fibre (cellulose, lignin) which adds bulk and softens the motions, thus preventing constipation. Other types of fibre, principally those in oats, rice, legumes, fruit and vegetables are soluble (pectin, gums). They lower cholesterol and affect the absorption of sugar, resulting in a moderate but sustained increase in blood sugar. Interestingly, they have little effect on bowel function, and similarly insoluble fibre does not affect blood cholesterol or sugar. It is therefore important to eat a variety of foods in order to obtain the full benefit from all the different types of dietary fibres.

It is advisable to gradually introduce foods containing fibre into the diet, as this will minimize flatulence. Bran can be eaten raw (one to two tablespoons), but is often more palatable in wholemeal bread and when sprinkled on other cereals. People who have eating and chewing difficulties can add bran to stewed fruit and use it in recipes. Drinking six to eight glasses of water each day is also necessary, as the fibre absorbs water to form softer bulkier motions. In addition fruit and vegetables should be consumed for their fibre content, with some being eaten raw and unpeeled. It is preferable to obtain fibre from a wholesome diet than take it in the form of tablets or as a powder.

Fibre and Disease

There are a number of problems associated with the low fibre diet eaten by many Australians. As previously mentioned, disorders of the bowel such as constipation, diverticulitis (inflamed pockets in the colon), haemorrhoids and bowel cancer can be treated and prevented by eating foods that are high in fibre. In addition cholesterol, heart disease, diabetes, obesity and the development of gall stones are all affected by dietary fibre. Again, moderation is necessary, as excess fibre is associated with the loss of certain nutrients such as calcium, iron and zinc.

TABLE 4.1 Fibre content of food (Australian Nutrition Foundation)

Food	Average serving	Approx. weight of serving	Grams of fibre per serving
Bread			
White,	1 slice	30 g	0.8
Mixed grain,	1 slice	30 g	1.5
Brown,	1 slice	30 g	1.5
Wholemeal,	1 slice	30 g	2.0
Cereals			
All bran,	$\frac{1}{2}$ cup	30 g	7.5
Bran [wheat],	2 tbsp	7 g	3.0
Rolled oats [cooked]	1 cup	250 g	3.3
Vita brits,	2	32 g	2.4
Wholemeal pasta [cooked]	1 cup	200 g	10.8
Vegetables			
Beans, French	$\frac{1}{3}$ cup	60 g	1.9
Beans, baked in tomato sauce	1 small can	110–130 g	8–9.5
Beans, kidney canned	$\frac{1}{2}$ cup	100 g	4.0
Broccoli, cooked	1 stalk	80 g	3.3
Carrot, raw	1 medium	100 g	2.8
Lettuce	2 leaves	25 g	0.4
Peas	$\frac{1}{3}$ cup	60 g	3.2
Potatoes, boiled in skin	1 medium	100 g	1.5
Tomato	1 medium	100 g	1.5
Fruit			
Apple with skin	1 medium	100 g	2.3
Apricots, dried	6 halves	25 g	6.0
Banana	1 medium	70 g	2.4
Grapes	1 small bunch	100 g	0.9
Orange	1 medium	100 g	2.0
Prunes	6	50 g with seed	6.7
Raisins	$\frac{1}{2}$ cup	75 g	5.1
Sultanas	$\frac{1}{2}$ cup	75 g	5.3

There are a number of reasons why fibre helps prevent constipation. As noted, it absorbs water causing the motions to be bulkier and softer. As a result the residue progresses more rapidly through the bowel and is expelled before the water can be reabsorbed. The normal bowel bacteria multiply well in the roughage. This further increases its bulk and results in the production of gases, both of which cause a more rapid expulsion of the motions. With softer stools there is less straining and haemorrhoids are prevented. In the case of bowel cancer it is similarly postulated that the more rapid passage through the bowel shortens the time it is exposed to cancer-producing substances. The greater amount of water in the motion will also tend to dilute these substances. The fibre may also alter the type of bacteria in the bowel so that the bile salts, which have been implicated in the development of bowel cancer, are metabolized.

Recent interest has been focused on the effects of fibre on blood cholesterol and sugar levels. The soluble fibre in fruit, vegetables, oats and legumes slows the absorption of sugar, which satisfies hunger for longer. Fibre also gives a feeling of fullness, because it remains in the stomach for a longer time. These factors are important in preventing obesity. The soluble fibres lower cholesterol by attaching to the cholesterol in the food and carrying it out of the body. Similarly the fibre binds to the bile salts which are produced in the liver from cholesterol. To replace the bile salts eliminated with the fibre the liver removes more cholesterol from the blood. The amounts of fibre required to achieve these effects is high, so it is advisable not to rely on fibre alone to lower cholesterol, but to also include low fat foods in the diet.

Protein

All the tissues and organs of the body are built from protein. In later life the protein in food is used by the body to repair and replace tissue protein that has been damaged as a result of either disease or ageing. Meat, fish, milk and eggs, are excellent dietary sources of protein with a number of vegetables also containing significant amounts. Important sources of vegetable protein are legumes, nuts and cereal products such as bread.

Protein is made up of a number of smaller components called amino acids. Meat products contain all the essential amino acids, but each vegetable is usually deficient in at least one. It is therefore important for vegetarians to combine various vegetables in order to obtain all the necessary amino acids. People sometimes embrace a vegetarian diet by simply excluding meat, without investigating which foods should be eaten to ensure all the necessary nutrients are retained in their diet. At the other extreme, if too much animal protein is eaten, this can contribute to a loss of calcium in the urine, which results in osteoporosis.

Fat

People of all ages have become increasingly health conscious, and no area has received more attention than the fat and cholesterol content of food. Indeed, this has already been reflected by a decrease in the consumption of eggs and meat. This section will explain the present state of knowledge in this rapidly expanding area and the findings of some exciting recent research.

A high fat and protein diet is associated with increased affluence. This has been linked with the increased incidence of a number of diseases, notably heart disease, diabetes, obesity and certain cancers (bowel and breast). It is therefore important to know the dietary sources of the various fats and how they can be reduced or modified to prevent these diseases developing.

Fats are a necessary part of nutrition but problems arise when they are eaten in excess. They have important functions in the body including the manufacture of some of the body's hormones (sex hormones and cortisol) as well as in the structure of cell walls. They are also involved in the absorption of fat soluble vitamins (vitamins A, D, E and K). Fat is often what makes food taste good, but it has almost double the kilojoules of protein and carbohydrates.

There are three types of fat in food: saturated, polyunsaturated and monounsaturated. This refers to the number (or saturation) of hydrogen atoms contained in each molecule of fat.

Saturated Fats

Animal foods are high in saturated fats and tend to raise blood cholesterol levels. Two plant based oils, coconut and palm oil, also contain saturated fats. This is important to keep in mind as they are frequently used in processed food such as cakes, biscuits, pies and fried foods. Chocolate is high in saturated fats, and it is this rather than the sugar that is most harmful to health.

Polyunsaturated Fats

These are usually vegetable oils. Polyunsaturated margarine, safflower, sunflower, cottonseed and grapeseed oils are all polyunsaturated products that are readily available. They should be used when fat is required, as they lower blood cholesterol levels. The omega-3 oils in fish have many interesting properties and are the subject of much research. They are dealt with later, on pages 98–9.

Monounsaturated Fats

Olive and canola oil have a high monounsaturated fat content. It is also present in peanut oil, peanuts, almonds and olives but in smaller amounts. Although avocado is cholesterol free, it contains significant amounts (20 per cent) of monounsaturated fat, and is one of the few fruits that contains fat. Monounsaturated fats have a beneficial effect on blood cholesterol levels. This is believed to explain the lower incidence of heart disease in Italy and Greece, countries where people have traditionally included olive oil as part of their diet.

Cholesterol

Cholesterol is a word that has become synonymous with unhealthy foods. It does however have a number of important physiological functions and interestingly more cholesterol is produced by the body than is obtained from food. After being manufactured in the liver, cholesterol is used in the production of hormones, bile acids (for digestion) and cell walls. Additional amounts of cholesterol are obtained from the diet, but this only represents 15 per cent of the total blood cholesterol.

The notoriety of cholesterol has been achieved by its recognition as one of the risk factors in heart disease. High levels of cholesterol in the blood result in it being deposited on the walls of the arteries. As the fat accumulates the body adds other substances (fibrous tissue, platelets and calcium), which gradually narrow the vessel. This process is called atherosclerosis, or hardening of the arteries. When this occurs in the arteries to the heart, blood flow to this vital organ is reduced and angina can occur. If there is complete blockage of the artery by fatty deposits the person suffers a heart attack.

Cholesterol is transported around the body in the bloodstream, but, being a fat, is insoluble in water. It must therefore attach to carriers called lipoproteins, and as the name suggests, these consist of cholesterol (fat or lipid) and protein. Some are light, and are called low density lipoproteins (LDL), while others are heavier, and are called high density lipoproteins (HDL). Each has a different function in controlling the accumulation of cholesterol in the arteries. The LDL carry the cholesterol to be deposited in the artery, while the HDL perform the opposite function, removing the cholesterol from the artery and carrying it back to the liver. This removal is beneficial, and therefore high levels of HDL mean more cholesterol is being cleared. HDL could loosely be termed 'good' cholesterol. The advantage of producing high levels of HDL may be inherited. There are some people who remain healthy, despite eating many fatty foods. This protection is probably due to the beneficial effects of the HDL. These substances can now be measured, and it has been shown that they are a better predictor of heart disease than total blood cholesterol level.

Measuring Blood Fats

Blood fats are measured to determine the risk of a person developing heart disease. Research has shown that a 1 per cent drop in cholesterol will result in a 2 per cent reduction in the risk of heart disease. It needs to be emphasized, however, that dietary fats are only one of the risk factors, and that obesity, high blood pressure, lack of exercise and stress should also be considered as part of a comprehensive approach to prevention.

The two most commonly measured fats in the blood are cholesterol and triglycerides. *Cholesterol* can be measured without fasting. Levels below 5.5 mmol/l are recommended by the National Heart Foundation. In later life although this relationship still exists it is not as dramatic as in younger years, which may influence the type of treatment chosen if cholesterol levels remain elevated. When measuring the *triglyceride* level it is important that the person fast for twelve hours prior to the blood sample being taken, because foods causes the level of triglycerides to rise. Values above 2 mmol/l are associated with an increased risk of heart disease.

More recently HDL, and the HDL/LDL ratio, can be calculated, which more accurately reflects the risk of developing heart disease. There are a number of even more sophisticated measurements, but they are not required for the majority of people.

Reducing Blood Fats

Certain foods have been held up as being capable of reducing blood fat levels. At present oat bran, fish oil and garlic are topical, with a number of claims as to their ability to lower cholesterol. These will be discussed, but it is also advisable that a broader view of the problem be taken, and the following suggestions adopted:

- Maintain an ideal weight — Those who are overweight would lower both the levels of cholesterol and triglycerides with weight reduction. This can be achieved by reducing the number of kilojoules eaten, as well as regularly performing moderate exercise.
- Fats — The total fat intake should be reduced and saturated fats replaced with polyunsaturated or monounsaturated fats. A lowering of cholesterol can also be achieved by reducing the intake of animal products and eating two to three fish or vegetarian meals per week.
- Fibre — The amount of wholegrain cereals and fruit and vegetables should be increased to replace high fat foods.
- Exercise — Regular exercise is important for all manner of problems, not least obesity. Refer back to Chapter 3 for detailed discussion of the benefits of increased physical activity.
- Alcohol — Excess alcohol can lead to elevated triglycerides and a host of other problems. A moderate amount of alcohol (one to two drinks per day) can be beneficial in preventing heart disease.
- Medication — Adopting a diet low in fats should result in

an average reduction in blood fats of 10 per cent. If the levels remain unacceptably high then medication may be prescribed. It is however important to note that the effect of cholesterol on heart disease in later life is not as pronounced as for younger age groups, and therefore perservering with a diet and further counselling from a doctor or dietician may be perferable. More research is required into the use of medication to treat high cholesterol in older people.

Most people focus on the cholesterol content of foods when attempting to reduce their blood cholesterol level. The main dietary sources of cholesterol are animal products, in particular egg yolk, liver, kidney and prawns. Those with high cholesterol should reduce their intake of these foods, for example, one to two eggs per week. As previously explained much of the cholesterol is produced by the body itself and therefore reducing dietary cholesterol alone may not significantly lower cholesterol levels. It is more important to reduce the total intake of fat, in particular saturated fat. Dietary guidelines suggest that the total amount of fat in the diet be reduced from 40 per cent to 30 per cent, and no more than one third of this should be saturated fats. The remainder should be comprised of polyunsaturated and monounsaturated fats.

Fish Oils

The low incidence of heart disease in Greenland Eskimos led researchers to suggest that this may be due to the high content of whale blubber and fish in their diet. These sea foods contain polyunsaturated fats called omega-3 fatty acids which have a number of interesting properties. It has been demonstrated that they lower LDL cholesterol and triglycerides levels in the blood, and reduce blood pressure. The omega-3 fatty acids appear to be the most effective means to lower triglycerides and are now often prescribed for this purpose. In addition, they thin the blood by causing the clotting cells to be less 'sticky'. This inhibits the formation of clots that block arteries, which may be important in preventing heart attacks and stroke. The substances in fish oil also have a 'calming' effect on the heart muscle and prevent irregular beats from developing. The omega-3 fish oils also affect inflammation and immunity. Research is still being undertaken on these important group of fats, and until more is known about possible side effects, they should not be taken in a concentrated form (for example in capsules) as a means of preventing disease. What can be recommended is two to three fish meals each week, as this has been shown to offer some protection against heart disease. The fish can be fresh, frozen or canned. Another source of omega-3 fatty acids is canola oil.

Oat Bran

Following the publication of Robert Kowalski's *The 8-week Cholesterol Cure* the sale of oat bran has sky-rocketed. It lowers cholesterol in the same way as the other cereals and fruits that contain soluble fibre. To achieve a significant reduction (14 per cent) a heaped cup of bran must be eaten, but often this is more than most people could normally tolerate. Oat bran and preferably whole oats should be included as part of a balanced diet, in which other cereals and fruits are eaten and the consumption of dietary fat reduced.

Garlic and Onion

Garlic and onion are known to reduce the level of blood fats. They also tend to slow blood clotting. Again it is wise to include them in a balanced diet, particularly to replace salt as a means of flavouring food. It is better to use fresh garlic in cooking than to buy garlic tablets.

The Pritikin Diet

Nathan Pritikin was an American nutritionist who formulated a diet after he became aware of his own heart problem and elevated cholesterol. The diet aims to dramatically decrease all fats consumed, reduce protein and salt, while substantially increasing the amount of carbohydrates eaten. It is an extremely strict diet but is effective in reducing weight as well as lowering cholesterol levels and blood pressure. Many people find this diet too severe and opt for what is called the 'modified' Pritikin, where the principles are followed but the restrictions relaxed.

Vitamins and Minerals

Vitamins and minerals, or 'micronutrients', are necessary for the body to function normally but are needed only in minute amounts. Some function as catalysts (substances used to facilitate chemical reactions) in cell metabolism, while others, notably calcium, are used structurally in the formation of bone. All the essential vitamins and minerals occur naturally in food and can be obtained by eating a nutritionally adequate diet.

Some elderly people are at risk of vitamin and mineral deficiency because, as previously discussed, decreased energy requirements can result in an inadequate intake of food. In addition, problems with health can adversely affect chewing and digestion, while practical considerations such as accessibility to shops and a limited income may restrict food shopping. The institutionalized elderly are at particular risk of having these deficiencies, as are ill or very stressed people. In certain circumstances a vitamin supplement may be indicated, but it is advisable to consult a doctor rather than to self-prescribe. As a general rule it is preferable to obtain all the nutrients from food, rather than rely on tablets to compensate for an inadequate diet.

There has been much interest in these nutrients as a means of treating and preventing diseases. Vitamin C has long been suggested as a 'cure' for the common cold, and more recently as a preventive against cancer. There are possible hazards in taking high doses of some vitamins, however. It is incorrect to believe that because they are 'natural', vitamins cannot be harmful. The amounts suggested are often many times the body's normal requirements, and are best considered as drug dosages. The prolonged intake of high doses of vitamin C has been associated with kidney stones, while vitamin A can cause skin problems if taken in large amounts.

There are thirteen vitamins and a number of minerals needed by the body, but only those which are particularly important in later life, or which influence common diseases, will be discussed here.

TABLE 4.2 Common sources of vitamins and minerals

Vitamin/Mineral	Common food source
Vitamin A	liver, dairy food, fish oil, dark green vegetables, yellow-orange fruit and vegetables
Vitamin B1*	wholegrain cereals, bread, yeast extract (vegemite, marmite, promite)
Vitamin B12	eggs, meat, liver
Vitamin C*	citrus fruits, tomatoes, potatoes, green vegetables
Vitamin D*	sunlight — most important source, dairy products, eggs, tinned fish (oil)
Vitamin E	vegetable oils, vegetables and fruit
Folic Acid*	green leafy vegetables (cabbage), fruit, liver
Calcium	milk products, green vegetables, sardines
Iron*	red meat, liver, chicken, breakfast cereals, vegetables
Potassium	apricots, banana, tomatoes, meat, whole grain cereals
Zinc	meat, vegetables, seafood
Selenium	cereals, meat

* Nutrients most likely to be deficient in older people

Vitamins

Vitamin A

Vitamin A is required for vision and for the maintenance of the skin and mucous membranes. It is a fat soluble vitamin and so is present in fish oil, liver and full fat dairy products. People on a low fat diet may therefore be at risk of being deficient in this vitamin.

Another source of vitamin A is beta-carotene, which is converted in the body to vitamin A. Yellow-orange fruit and vegetables, and green vegetables contain beta-carotene. Recent research has revealed that beta-carotene is associated with a lower incidence of lung and skin cancer. Adequate amounts of fruit and vegetables should be included in a healthy diet, although it is not advisable to take large quantities of beta-carotene, as this can cause yellow discolouration of the skin. It has been found that when vitamin A, in the form of Retin-A, is applied to the skin, some of the effects of skin ageing can be reversed.

The Vitamin B group

A deficiency of vitamin B1 (thiamin) is common in those who drink excessive amounts of alcohol. This can result in brain damage and mental illness. Thiamin can reverse some of these problems and is often taken by people participating in alcohol rehabilitation programmes.

Niacin (vitamin B3) has the interesting property of reducing blood cholesterol. The amount needed is many times the quantities found naturally in food and therefore the effect is better described as the result of a drug dose.

Vitamin B12 and folic acid deficiencies are occasionally present in later life and cause anaemia. Insufficient B12 in the body can also lead to a deterioration of the brain and nervous system. A lack of B12 is the result of the absence of a substance in the stomach (intrinsic factor) which enables B12 to be absorbed. Replacement is therefore by an injection every few months, as people with this deficiency cannot obtain the vitamin from food. Folic acid deficiency on the other hand is usually the result of poor diet and drinking too much alcohol. It can be corrected by eating green leafy vegetables.

Vitamin C

The ability of vitamin C to prevent disease was first suggested by Linus Pauling, who believed it 'cured' the common cold. Subsequent studies have revealed that while it does not stop a person from catching a cold, the severity of the symptoms may be reduced. More recently attention has focused on the role of vitamin C and other antioxidants in preventing cancer, but the doses used in these studies are significantly larger than the amounts naturally available in food. Until more information is available vitamin C cannot be endorsed as a cure for cancer, although these findings should not be ignored. A logical approach is to ensure that a balanced diet contains significant amounts of this important vitamin which is present in citrus fruits and vegetables, particularly cabbage and broccoli. Vitamin C is easily destroyed in the preparation of food (excessive cutting, cooking and by baking soda), so it is advisable to eat at least some of these foods raw.

Vitamin D

Vitamin D is unique in that it is produced by the body when the skin is exposed to sunlight. Older people who are housebound or in institutions are at risk of developing vitamin D deficiency if they never venture outdoors. In these cases it is important that dairy foods and tinned fish are eaten, since these are good dietary sources of vitamin D. This vitamin increases the amount of calcium absorbed from food and is involved in the formation of bone. A deficiency of vitamin D will aggravate osteoporosis.

Vitamin E

Vitamin E has excited much interest as an antioxidant, and has been loosely linked to the prevention of cancer, heart disease and retarding the ageing process. Again, more research needs to be undertaken to substantiate these claims. Deficiency of vitamin E is rare as it is present in many foods. Being a fat soluble vitamin, vegetable oils and margarine are particularly rich sources.

Retaining Vitamins in Food

A number of storage and cooking processes reduce the vitamin content of food, and the loss can be minimized by a number of simple adjustments to the practices of food storage and preparation. It is preferable to make smaller but more frequent purchases to ensure freshness of perishable foods such as fruit and vegetables. Refrigeration prolongs this freshness, with frozen vegetables able to be stored for long periods without their vitamins being destroyed. It is also advisable to cook frozen vegetables immediately, rather than allowing them to thaw. Excessive cutting of foods, or allowing them to soak and stand for a long time, also results in the loss of vitamins. Vegetables should be cooked for the shortest possible time and using the least amount of water. The remaining water contains vitamins which can be used as a basis for soups and other dishes. Steaming and microwave cooking are excellent methods of cooking vegetables, while adding bicarbonate of soda and cooking in copper saucepans destroys the vitamins.

Minerals

Calcium

An adequate intake of calcium is important for bone structure and the proper functioning of muscles and nerves. Osteoporosis is a common problem in later life, particularly in women after menopause. It is partly due to a deficiency of calcium. The enthusiasm to lower cholesterol and reduce weight has unfortunately resulted in people consuming less dairy products, which are high in calcium. Many of these foods are now available with low or reduced fat content (and some even have added calcium), so they can be safely eaten by people watching their fat intake.

Osteoporosis is prevented by consuming adequate amounts of calcium *throughout* life. After menopause the recommended intake is 1000 mg per day. This is well above the average 500–700 mg that most people take in. The foods richest in calcium are dairy products such as milk, cheeses and yoghurt. (Butter and cream contain almost no calcium.) In addition fish, particularly canned fish with bones (sardines), and green vegetables contain smaller but valuable quantities of calcium.

A simple rule to ensure an adequate intake of calcium is to have two 'serves' of dairy produce each day, with one serve being equivalent to a large glass (300 ml) of milk. Thus two glasses of milk, or one glass of milk and forty grams of yellow cheese, will satisfy the body's daily requirement. It must be emphasized that this is in addition to a normal healthy diet that contains other sources of calcium. Two serves of dairy produce plus the smaller quantities of calcium in other foods will bring the total to 1000 mg per day. If this amount is not consumed then calcium supplements may be required, but food sources are preferable. The table on the following page lists the calcium content of some foods.

Iron

Iron plays an important part in the formation of red blood cells. It is not uncommon for iron deficiency to be present in an older person due to blood loss, chronic disease or an inadequate diet. Meat is an excellent source of iron, and is better absorbed than the iron present in vegetables. It is therefore important for vegetarians to eat sufficient quantities of eggs, green vegetables, lentils and fortified breakfast cereals to obtain the iron they need. There is some evidence to suggest that iron deficiency increases the incidence of stomach and bowel cancer.

TABLE 4.3 Calcium content of food (Department of Health, NSW)

Food	Average portion	Calcium (mg)
Milk	300 ml	335
Skim Milk	300 ml	348
Modified milk [Hi-Lo]	300 ml	408
Low fat modified milk [Shape]	300 ml	468
Yoghurt, plain	200 g	380
Cheese, cheddar type	40 g	300
Cottage cheese	40 g	20–25
Ice cream	150 ml	100
Cream	20 g	12
Butter	20 g	2
Fish, cooked	100 g	25
Salmon, canned with bones	100 g	95
Sardines, canned	50 g	250
Egg, one	55 g	25
Haricot or lima beans, cooked, $\frac{1}{2}$ cup	100 g	50
Tahini, 1 tablespoon	20 g	180
Bread, 1 slice white, brown, wholemeal	30 g	10
Oatmeal, cooked, 1 cup	250 g	15
Cornflakes, 1 cup	30 g	1
Wheat breakfast biscuits, 2	30 g	10
Vegetables, cooked,		
Broccoli	100 g	75
Parsley	10 g	30
Fruit, average, raw, 1 piece	100 g	10
Figs, dried	50 g	140

Potassium

'Fluid tablets' (diuretics) are prescribed to treat high blood pressure and kidney and heart disease. A common problem with these medications is the loss of potassium in the urine. Usually a potassium supplement is prescribed, but occasionally, if the diuretic is not strong, attention to the dietary intake of potassium may suffice. Apricots, bananas, tomatoes, meat and whole grain cereals are all good sources of potassium. It is advisable to check with a doctor before ceasing potassium tablets and relying on diet alone.

Sodium

Most Australians eat food which has an excessively high salt (sodium) content, and the amount of salt consumed increases with age. This significantly contributes to high blood pressure. If not detected and treated, high blood pressure can lead to strokes, heart disease and kidney disease. Most health authorities advise that the amount of salt in the diet be reduced in order to prevent these problems. Not everyone on a high salt diet will develop high blood pressure, and those people with a family history of the problem are at most risk. As there are no other criteria by which to assess whose blood pressure will rise, it is advisable for everyone to reduce their salt intake.

Salt is necessary for regulating the amount of water in the body, and for the normal functioning of nerves and muscles. Adequate amounts are obtained naturally from foods such as meat, eggs and milk. Three quarters of the salt eaten has been added to food and is not required by the body. Processed and snack foods are the most common sources of this unnecessary salt. In addition it is 'hidden' in foods such as biscuits and bread that often do not taste salty. The salt in cooking ingredients such as monosodium glutamate (MSG) and baking soda (sodium bicarbonate) complicates the problem of knowing which foods to exclude in order to lower the intake of salt.

A low salt diet prevents fluid retention and people may notice a weight loss of one to two kilograms. A low salt diet also ensures that more calcium is retained by the body, thus contributing in a small way to preventing osteoporosis. A person with high blood pressure should discuss with their doctor a trial of non-drug treatment, including a low salt diet, weight loss and stress management. This is often all that is needed to lower mildly elevated blood pressure in an older person. Even if medication is necessary, the dose required should be lower if these measures are implemented. An interesting relationship exists between sodium (salt) and potassium, and their effect on blood pressure. In addition to reducing the total intake of salt there is evidence that a higher ratio of potassium relative to sodium in the diet may help prevent high blood pressure. Many fruit and vegetables have a high proportion of potassium to sodium but this is reduced when the food is processed. Manufacturing tomato sauce from tomatoes is one example of a food that has natural protective properties being converted to a high salt containing product.

Two of the most obvious ways to reduce salt intake are not to add it to cooking or at the table. This is preferably done gradually; initially the food may taste bland, but once the taste buds have 'readjusted', the true flavours in food not disguised by salt will be discovered. Some other suggestions for lowering salt intake include:

- Reduce the amount of salt used in cooking;
- Avoid adding salt at the table either directly or 'hidden' in sauces and pickles;
- Limit foods with high salt content: sausages, salami, olives, smoked foods, snack foods e.g. salted nuts and chips;
- Check labels and choose those foods that have low salt or are salt-free e.g. bread, butter, margarine, soups, sauces;
- Add flavour to food with lemon juice, spices and herbs (garlic, pepper);
- Drink low salt (sodium) mineral water (less than 50 mg per litre);
- Avoid cooking ingredients that contain sodium; MSG, baking soda.

Zinc

This mineral is mentioned as studies have shown that it is occasionally deficient in people who are institutionalized. Lack of zinc causes wounds to heal slowly and the loss of taste. As a result the appetite is reduced, which further aggravates the deficiency. Zinc is present in liver, meat, legumes, green leafy vegetables and oysters.

Selenium

This little known mineral is an antioxidant, and is commonly mentioned with vitamin E as being associated with a lower incidence of cancer. More work needs to be done before the significance of these findings can be applied in any practical way. Selenium is obtained from cereals and meat, and reflects the selenium levels of the soil in which the food has been grown. Selenium supplements should not be taken, as excessive amounts of this mineral can be extremely toxic.

Water

This vital nutrient, without which life could not exist, should not be overlooked. The body is comprised mostly of water and six to eight glasses of water each day are required to replace the fluids that are lost mainly through perspiration and in the urine. It is preferable to drink water rather than soft drinks and alcohol, as it is 'cleansing' and totally free of kilojoules.

Those in later life experience less thirst, and therefore must be aware of the need to increase their fluid intake in hot weather and during illness. Extra fluids are required particularly if a fever or diarrhoea is present. Dehydration is even more serious if a person is on medication. The drugs become more concentrated and in extreme cases a build-up to dangerous levels can occur. Fluids during the meal can also aid chewing, as saliva production decreases with age.

HEALTHY DIETARY GUIDELINES

Many older people were brought up to believe that butter, cream, meat and eggs were wholesome and healthy. Potatoes, bread and other 'starchy' foods, on the other hand, were considered 'fattening'. There have been significant advances in our understanding of nutrition and this has caused revolutionary changes in our attitude to many foods. Despite these changes, however, many people continue to consume a diet that is high in fat, sugar and salt, but low in starch and fibre. As has been noted, this contributes to the development of a number of diseases, including heart disease and cancer. In order to improve the health of the whole community, the Australian Government commissioned a report, which recommended certain dietary guidelines. These are as follows:

- Choose a nutritious diet from a variety of foods;
- Control your weight;
- Avoid eating too much fat;
- Avoid eating too much sugar;
- Eat more bread and cereals (preferably wholegrain), fruit and vegetables;
- Limit alcohol consumption;
- Use less salt;
- Drink more water.

These are recommendations for healthy eating and not

weight loss. Some people may, however, lose weight if they adopt this eating plan, due to the reduction in the energy value of the food consumed.

Planning a Menu

It is necessary to translate all the information contained in this chapter into a practical meal plan. To allow for individual variation in taste and different cultural habits, the suggestions are fairly broad. Although the recommendations are mainly for active, healthy older people, they also form the basis for diabetic, low fat and weight reduction diets. In these special circumstances, it is wise to consult a doctor or dietician to ensure adequate nutrition is maintained while the diet is modified to deal with the medical problem.

The 1,2,3,4,5+ Nutrition Plan has been developed by the CSIRO Division of Human Nutrition, to serve as a food guide for people who wish to eat a healthy and balanced diet. It

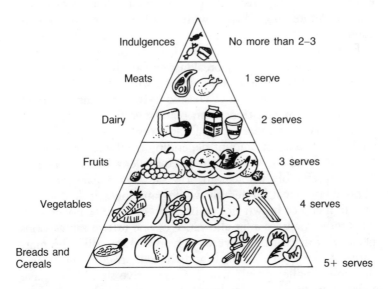

FIGURE 4.2 The food pyramid according to the 1,2,3,4,5+ Nutrition Plan.

contains adequate amounts of nutrients but is not high in kilojoules. The numbers refer to the serves per day of each food group:

> 5 or more serves — cereals and breads
> 4 serves — vegetables
> 3 serves — fruit
> 2 serves — dairy produce
> 1 serve — meat and alternatives
> + indulgences and fats (no more than two or three)

Bread and Cereals

These foods include breads of which there are now many different varieties. Wholemeal, brown and mixed grain breads are preferable as they contain more dietary fibre, vitamins and minerals. Salt free or low salt loaves are also available. Bread itself is not 'fattening'. It is usually what is eaten with the bread (butter, jam, honey) that contains most of the fat and kilojoules. Buying unsliced bread allows thicker slices to be cut, therefore more bread with relatively. less 'topping' is eaten.

Pasta, rice, noodles and breakfast cereals are all in this category. There are many breakfast cereals available and it is important to read the labels to check which have the lowest fat, salt and sugar content. Toasted muesli contains more of these unhealthy additions than plain muesli.

Five serves or more of bread and cereal should be eaten each day, the exact amount depending on the amount of activity undertaken. One serve is equivalent to one slice of bread, (preferably wholegrain, low salt, low sugar), one cup of breakfast cereal (preferably wholegrain, low salt, low sugar), or half a cup of brown rice or one cup of pasta (wholegrain). This serve includes a fat allowance of one to two tablespoons per day of margarine, olive or polyunsaturated oil. The margarine to be used on bread, and the oils in cooking or as a dressing. Smaller people who are less active should not have more than five serves of bread or cereal and should reduce their fat allowance to one tablespoon per day.

Vegetables

Vegetables are ideal foods to 'fill up' on; they are low in fat and high in many important nutrients. It is worth developing the habit of eating these foods as snacks, instead of processed foods which are less healthy. As many of the vitamins are destroyed by cooking, it is important that some vegetables are eaten raw or only lightly cooked. Choose those that are in season, as they are unlikely to have been stored, and will therefore taste better and be more nutritious. Food in season is also more reasonably priced.

Ensure a variety of vegetables are eaten, as each has different nutrients. At least one serve should come from each of the starchy, dark green leafy, red-yellow and other types of vegetables. Of the starchy vegetables, one serve should equal one medium potato, a third of a cup of parsnip, or half a medium sweet potato. One serve of the red-yellow vegetables, such as carrot or pumpkin, should be about a third of a cup. A third of a cup of dark green leafy and other vegetables also equals one serve.

Fruit

Fruit can be eaten raw, stewed, canned (avoid syrup) or dried. Fruit juice is not included as it does not contain fibre or bulk. If fruit is not eaten more serves of vegetables can be eaten, as they contain the same level of nutrients as fruit. However, if vegetables are not eaten it is not possible to replace them with fruit, as fruit alone will not supply all the essential nutrients.

One serve of fruit equals one medium apple, orange or banana; three stone fruits such as apricots or plums; ten to twelve grapes or berry fruits; four to six pieces of dried fruit, or a third of a cup of stewed or canned fruit.

Dairy Foods

The extra calcium needed to prevent osteoporosis has led to a greater intake of dairy produce being recommended in later life. Where possible low fat dairy foods should be chosen.

One serve equals one large glass or small carton of milk (300 ml), 40 gm cheese, or 200 gm carton of plain or fruit yoghurt. Cottage and ricotta cheeses are not included here, as they contain only small amounts of calcium.

Non-dairy alternatives that are equivalent to 300 ml of milk are: 1500 ml soy milk, or 300 ml of calcium fortified soy milk.

Meat and Alternatives

Lean red meat is a source of protein which also contains important nutrients such as iron and zinc. It is necessary to choose lean cuts of meat and trim off excess fat. The meat can be grilled, baked or microwaved without the addition of extra fat. It is acceptable to have a double serve of red meat every other day instead of one serve each day.

Poultry, fish, eggs and legumes can be substituted for meat, particularly if people have high energy needs. There is increasing evidence that eating fish can have a beneficial effect on health and reduce the risk of heart disease, however, many of these advantages are lost if it is fried. Legumes are another valuable source of protein. They include soya, lima, kidney, butter and mung beans, and chickpeas and lentils. One serve of cooked lean meat should equal 60 gm, a serve of chicken (no skin) or fish should weigh 120 gm. Two thirds of a cup of legumes equal one serve, as does two eggs.

Indulgences

This group of foods have little nutritional value and are by no means essential for survival. Biscuits, cakes, soft drinks and alcohol are best avoided, however the reality of the western diet is that these are commonly eaten. The best option is therefore to limit the amount of these indulgences to no more than one to two per day, and wherever possible to replace them with extra serves of breads, fruit, vegetables or dairy products.

One serve equals: two standard glasses of alcoholic drink, soft drink or cordial; one medium piece of cake or bun; one tablespoon of fat spreads or oils; three to four tablespoons of single cream; two to three biscuits; 30 gm chocolate, toffees or nuts; 60 gm jam or honey, and 40 gm table sugar (eight teaspoons).

Take away foods such as pies, pasties and chips are equivalent to three serves of these foods.

5 STRESS AND RELAXATION

'A sound mind in a sound body.'
Juvenal

A vital part of total good health is mental tranquillity and emotional happiness. Threats and challenges have always been part of the human experience, with survival determined by the ability to cope with and adapt to these changes. The pressures of modern living have resulted in an increase in the amount of stress experienced by people of all ages.

Stress is usually a change that challenges or threatens a person's wellbeing. It is a combination of the cause of the stress (stressor) and the individual's response to it. Stressors can be events in the outside environment such as retirement or moving home. They can also be personal problems like ill health. Even thoughts can be stressful. The amount of discomfort a person experiences depends on his or her perception of and ability to cope with a stressor. Retirement may be welcomed by some people as relief from an unsatisfying job, while others, who have no desire to stop working, may find it very stressful.

There is a general misconception that stress is always negative and unpleasant. In fact some degree of stress is normal and at times even desirable. It can motivate people to succeed and improve their performance, for example. A complete absence of stress is associated with apathy, inactivity and a lack of ambition. Problems arise when the amount of stress is overwhelming or continues for a prolonged period of time. In these circumstances people are overloaded with pressure. They experience feelings of strain and anxiety which may cause a decrease in performance. These negative aspects of stress, more accurately termed distress, are those usually implied when the word is used in everyday speech. A broader, more balanced view of stress, appreciating the desirable as well as its unpleasant aspects, allows a person to understand and cope better with the challenges of life.

It is incorrect to assume that only excessive work and pressure from a hectic lifestyle result in anxiety. Inactivity and boredom can also lead to distressing feelings of uselessness. Studying stress in animals has revealed some interesting results. Those subjected to a moderate amount of stress lived longer than the animals that experienced either no stress or frequent and severe stress. These results may also apply to humans — a moderate or optimal amount of stress is likely to be beneficial and contribute to a robust active later life.

Everything a person does in life has the potential to be stressful, particularly if it is associated with change. Of course adjustments are not always detrimental. Remarriage and embarking on a new career are both stressful but can have positive consequences. In order to gain rewards, it is necessary to take calculated risks. On the other hand, negative events, such as the death of a spouse, are distressing experiences that are associated with intense feelings of sadness and grief.

The individual's interpretation and reaction to such experiences determines how stressful they will turn out to be. The same situation can be viewed by one person as unpleasant and dreadful, while by another as a stimulating challenge. Mature 'children' leaving home can be regarded by parents to be a desirable part of normal development and independence, the culmination of successful parenting. It can also be viewed negatively, as an event which leaves parents feeling abandoned and alone. Likewise, the process of ageing can be viewed with anxiety and dread, as the 'end of life', whereas many opportunities and challenges remain if an alternative, more positive approach is adopted. People react differently to the same situation, viewing it either positively as a challenge, or negatively as a threat or loss. Those who face problems optimistically are less likely to suffer from the unpleasant effects of stress.

Stressful thoughts can also arise by anticipating problems, and by imagining a worse outcome than will probably occur.

For example, if the presence of a relatively minor symptom leads to the unrealistic conclusion that this may be due to a life threatening disease, feelings of distress and anxiety are increased. Such over-reaction is the result of negative thoughts and is unrelated to the seriousness of the illness. The uncertainty of impending changes, which may not be within a person's control, can also result in anxiety. Those who voluntarily retire have more control over their lives and are less likely to feel anxious than a colleague who is unwillingly forced to stop work. The same event can have opposite emotional effects as the result of different attitudes.

Self-talk is a term used to describe the internal thoughts that everyone experiences. As we can see, stress is frequently the result of negative self-talk. In regards to older people, examples of negative self-talk are:

- 'I am too old to be useful.'
- 'It is normal at my age to have arthritis in the knee.'
- 'Why bother about leading a healthy life at my age.'

Of course these thoughts may become self-fulfilling prophecies, for if the expectations for later life are low it is unlikely that people will strive to alter their outcome. Taking the above examples, a person who engages in positive self-talk is likely to view the same problems from an entirely different perspective:

- 'I have a great deal of experience and wisdom which is useful to other people.'
- 'My other knee is the same age as the painful one, so it is not normal. I will find out what the problem is and how it can be remedied.'
- 'I am a worthwhile person and deserve to look after myself.'

Positive self-talk can entirely change a situation. It often leads to action, rather than gloomy acceptance and passivity. People who engage in positive self-talk are likely to have high self-esteem. They endeavour to retain control over their lives, while remaining open to alternative ideas. Moving to different accommodation, for example, is less stressful if the control for this decision remains with the person affected. Enforced relocation by family and friends is a frequent cause of distress in older people, and can be avoided if individuals insist that their own wishes are fulfilled.

Response to stress is determined by past experiences, personality and the ability to cope with problems. Contrary to expectations, older adults generally cope well in times of stress. This can be due to their greater experience in dealing with life's difficulties. Their maturity also offers a philosophical perspective from which to view life's changes.

STRESS IN LATER LIFE

There are three broad sources of stress in later life. They range from everyday hassles through to important life events, and include chronic causes of stress. Each contributes to the overall amount of stress experienced by an individual.

Chronic stress has usually been present for a long period of time and is not unique to later life. Financial hardship and an unhappy marriage are examples. Negative self-talk and low self-esteem can cast a pessimistic shadow over all of life's events, and if this is the case can also lead to chronic stress. Unrealistic expectations and a perfectionist attitude are other factors that increase stress, as the individual strains to perform beyond reasonable limits. There is no reason to accept negative attitudes and feelings as permanent simply because they have been present for a long time. The individual must be willing to work towards changing negative attitudes, and some of the ways this can be done are looked at later in this chapter.

Everyday hassles are those minor, irritating annoyances that intrude on most people's lives. Traffic delays, waiting in queues and misplacing things can be frustrating, but are not usually distressing. Unfortunately, however, those under stress from other pressures can over-react to these small events. It is important to recognize and focus on resolving the *real* source of the stress, rather than be deceived into believing that a superficial hassle is the main problem.

Life events are significant experiences that are likely to change or have an impact on a person's life. Forty-three such situations have been described by Holmes and Rahe, who rated them according to the amount of stress each would produce. The total 'stress score' over one year was then compared to the development of illness. They suggested that the more stress experienced the higher a person scored and the more likely they were to become physically ill.

TABLE 5.1 The Holmes-Rahe scale of recent experiences

Death of a spouse	100
Divorce	73
Marital separation	65
Jail term	63
Death of close family member	63
Personal injury or illness	53
Marriage	50
Fired at work	47
Marital reconciliation	45
Retirement	45
Change in health of family member	44
Sexual difficulties	39
Gain of new family member	39
Business readjustment	39
Change in financial state	38
Death of a close friend	37
Change to different work	36
Change in number of arguments with spouse	35
Mortgage over $10 000	31
Foreclosure on mortgage or loan	30
Change in responsibilities at work	29
Son or daughter leaving home	29
Trouble with in-laws	29
Outstanding personal achievements	28
Wife begins or stops working	26
Change in living conditions	25
Change in residence	20
Change in recreation	19
Change in church activities	19
Change in social activities	18
Mortgage loan less than $10 000	17
Change in sleeping habits	16
Change in number of family get-togethers	15
Change in eating habits	15
Vacation	13
Christmas	12
Minor violations of the law	11

Total the number of stressful events that have occurred in the previous twelve months. If the score is above 200 then, according to this approach, there is a greater than average chance of developing symptoms of illness.

The Scale of Recent Experience is meant as a broad guide; naturally, individual responses to stressful events vary widely. Moreover, the table cannot take into account the impact of other pressures such as longstanding stress and worries. Some of these life events are positive and may actually improve health. Retirement, for example, can lead to an overall decrease in stress once the adjustment has been made. The Holmes-Rahe score is most beneficial if used as a 'warning' for an individual to start working towards maintaining good health.

The number of life events tends to decrease with advancing years. Those that do occur, however, tend to have a greater impact. The death of a spouse is an extremely distressing event and is generally faced later in life. Ageing itself requires a new self-image as youthful appearance wanes. Confronting problems such as bereavement and changes in physical appearance is the first crucial step towards resolution. People at any age can 'grow' and learn from their experiences.

THE STRESS RESPONSE

The body's reaction to a stressful situation is a survival response, a primitive reaction designed for protection. For primitive peoples the threat was usually physical, such as attack by a wild animal. The response alerted them to the emergency, so they could immediately react by either fighting or escaping. This is called the 'fight or flight response'.

There are a number of changes in bodily function associated with this reaction, and these occur unconsciously. Adrenalin and cortisone are released and surge through the body, preparing it to cope with the threat. Heart rate, blood pressure and breathing increase to meet the extra demands for blood and oxygen. The pupils dilate to improve vision so that the danger is clearly seen. Muscles tighten ready for action and blood is diverted away from other organs to supply the active muscles with nourishment. Stored sugar is released by the liver and serves as an added source of energy. An increased amount of blood also goes to the brain so that the person can remain alert and think quickly. To compensate for this, blood is channelled away from the skin and limbs, while sweat is produced to cool the body. These changes cause the person to look pale and have cold, clammy hands and feet. In anticipation of injury the blood clots more easily and there are changes in the immune system. During the crisis special hormones (endorphines) are released in the brain to relieve any pain that may be experienced as a result of damage to the body.

This response is intended as a brief automatic reaction to protect a person from physical danger. After the danger has passed it is important that the body return to its normal resting state. Fighting or fleeing, both of which are physical activities, consume the released adrenalin. This helps to complete the stress response and allows the body to regain its equilibrium. Using up the adrenalin during exercise explains the beneficial effect of increased activity in reducing stress. Relaxation also reverses the physical and emotional changes that occur as a result of stress.

Unfortunately the stresses of modern living differ significantly from those for which the stress response was originally intended. Today stress is often subtle and easily overlooked. The pace of modern life is hectic and many daily hassles, such as driving in heavy traffic, are accepted as normal while in fact being stressful. Problems can also continue unresolved for long periods of time, as occurs when a couple remains unhappily married for many years. Ill health, financial difficulties and misunderstandings with friends are other commonly encountered stresses. The conflicts are usually verbal or emotional; physically escaping from these types of problems will not lead to their resolution. Thought and logic are more likely to resolve today's problems.

As a result of these differences, the aforementioned physiological changes persist for prolonged periods of time. The body is in a constant state of readiness and on alert. There are no periods of rest, so that many of the biochemical and physical changes that were intended to be temporary become permanent. The cause of stress may not be obvious or is accepted as a part of everyday life, and therefore remains unresolved. Not surprisingly, this places significant strain on the body, and this may result in a number of problems and even disease.

STRESS AND ILLNESS

The suggestion that emotional and physical health are intimately related has been suspected for many years. In eastern cultures, where yoga and meditation are practised, this has been accepted for centuries. The phrase 'a healthy body — a healthy mind' has only recently been explained scientifically, and the physiological changes which occur in a person under pressure form the basis of this understanding. There are a multitude of symptoms that occur due to sustained or intense stress, and each is an amplification of the normal brief stress response. Table 5.2 illustrates the likely progression of the normal reactions to stress, extending to symptoms of prolonged stress and finally disease.

When a person is constantly 'on alert', she or he feels tense, restless and unable to unwind. Sleep disturbances are common as are lack of concentration and forgetfulness. Confidence is undermined, which results in indecision and confusion. As performance decreases there often is disorganization and frantic rushing from one task to another. Emotional outbursts are associated with negative feelings such as anger, irritability and fear. This in turn affects relationships with other people.

Physical signs of prolonged stress include persistent elevation of the blood pressure which may manifest itself as dizziness and headaches. Forceful beating of the heart is felt as palpitations which are often noticed while resting at night. Tight spasms in muscles, particularly around the neck, shoulders and lower back, can cause discomfort and pain in these areas. Indigestion, nausea and diarrhoea are the result of changes that occur in the digestive system. Tense people complain of increased perspiration and have cold, clammy hands and feet. The constant pressure is physically and emotionally exhausting, leaving a person worn out and tired.

Unfortunately the response to these warning signs may be inappropriate; for example, a person may turn to food or drugs for relief. Over-eating and obesity can be the result of stress, and alcohol, cigarettes and drugs may be consumed in the belief that they will relieve unpleasant feelings. This is incorrect — these unhealthy habits only compound the problem and contribute to ill health.

There is increasing evidence to suggest that stress can lead to the development of certain diseases, both directly as well as through an unhealthy lifestyle. The suppression of the immune system during times of stress is well documented and results in an increased incidence of infections. Although unproven, it has been suggested that as the surveillance and destruction of cancer cells is performed by the immune system, any factor that affects its normal functioning may allow a cancer to grow. Smoking and excessive alcohol intake, on the other hand, have been firmly linked with certain cancers.

The effect of stress on heart disease has been extensively studied. In the 1960s two American doctors, Rosenman and Friedman, psychologically assessed men who had suffered a heart attack to determine if their personality and ability to deal with stress could be linked to the development of heart disease. The doctors found that certain individuals, whom they termed 'Type A', were more likely to suffer from heart disease. These people tended to be impatient, competitive and ambitious. They were time conscious, always rushing to meet deadlines, and frequently aggressive. This was in contrast to the 'Type B' person who was less likely to have heart disease and tended to be relaxed, unhurried and non-competitive. In contributing to heart disease, stress was found to operate independently of the other factors such as smoking, overweight, cholesterol and exercise. Other doctors have not agreed with these findings and the subject remains controversial.

As noted, high blood pressure is also the result of sustained stress and if left untreated contributes to the development of heart attack and stroke. Arthritis, fibrositis, neckache and backache all have an emotional component, and allowing the muscles to relax often reduces the amount of pain experienced. Irritable bowel syndrome is another condition related to stress, and manifests itself as stomach pains with constipation or diarrhoea. Frequently decreased sexual interest is due to problems within a relationship or preoccupation with other worries.

The connection between stress and emotional illness is more obvious. Depression and anxiety are often the result of stress and frequently related to the losses which can occur in later life. Ill health, caring for loved ones and death are formidable adjustments for people of any age. Many of the

TABLE 5.2 Stress and Illness

a — Normal stress symptoms
b — Symptoms of prolonged stress
c — Associated disease

Brain

a Increased blood supply; pupils dilate; endorphines released to reduce pain; alert; hormones released that cause the adrenal gland to release adrenalin
b Tense; restless; disturbed sleep; reduced sex drive; change in appetite; smoking
c Anxiety; depression; interpersonal/relationship problems

Muscles

a Increased blood supply; muscles tighten ready for activity
b Tense aching muscles; neckache; backache
c Arthritis; fibrositis

Heart

a Increased heart rate; raised blood pressure
b Palpitations; headache; dizziness
c Heart disease (Type A personality); hypertension

Lungs

a Increased rate breathing
b Breathlessness
c Asthma

Adrenal

a Releases adrenalin and cortisone
b Altered immunity
c Increased incidence of infections, allergies, ?cancer

Digestive system

a Reduced activity and blood supply
b Nervous diarrhoea; indigestion
c Irritable bowel syndrome

Skin

a Sweat; blood diverted from skin to muscle and brain
b Cold, clammy skin; excessive sweating
c Skin rashes; itch

Genital and Urinary

a Blood diverted away from kidneys and genital organs
b Lack of interest in sex
c Sexual problems (largely the result of emotional problems)

problems encountered in later life cannot be altered, but the distress they cause can be reduced by a positive attitude, relaxation and the development of skills to cope with these situations.

IDENTIFYING STRESS

Individuals often do not recognize that they are subjected to excessive strain and pressure. The motivation to reduce stress must be preceded by an awareness that the problem exists. A number of stressful experiences are listed in the Holmes-Rahe scale, which provides a useful indicator of the strain an event may provoke. Ill health due to a heart attack can lead to feelings of anxiety and depression. Denial of these unpleasant emotions allows them to continue, while recognizing them is the first step towards resolution. After a heart attack seeking information about the type and frequency of exercise, resumption of sexual activity and when to start driving again, alleviates the anxiety induced by uncertainty and lack of knowledge. The stress from other events is sometimes unavoidable. Grief following bereavement is best allowed to proceed until the natural process of mourning is completed. Because a number of the experiences listed in the Holmes-Rahe scale normally affect an individual's life, their impact can be minimized by planning, and prompt action when these situations arise.

Stressful thoughts and feelings are more difficult to recognize, as they are often accepted as a normal part of an individual's personality. A busy lifestyle does not allow time for contemplation or analysis of inner thoughts and emotions. The body's warning signals are frequently ignored until they become serious. An increasingly severe tension headache and painful, tight neck muscles are common examples. Complaints such as these are dismissed or misinterpreted as physical ailments when in fact they reflect tension within the body. It is important to be consciously aware of these signals so that they can be relieved.

There are two simple techniques for recognizing hidden stress. The first is to search for tension by being aware of the state of one's own body and its inner emotions.

Exercise 1

Sit or lie comfortably. Loosen any tight clothing and close your eyes. Begin by becoming conscious of the chair or bed being in contact with your body. Feel it pressing. Hear the sounds around you. Concentrate on them. Now turn your attention to your own body. Focus on your head and neck. Is there any pain, or tightness in the muscles? Is your face frowning and jaw clenched? Gradually move around your body focusing on each individual part . . . chest . . . stomach . . . back . . . arms . . . legs . . . Become conscious of your breathing and heartbeat. Do not try to change the sensations, simply recognize what your body is experiencing.

Now turn to your innermost thoughts. Allow any feelings and emotions to enter your mind. Reflect on recent events and the sentiments they have provoked. Are they pleasant and satisfying or do they cause anxiety and anger? Allow the session to continue for as long as you feel comfortable. Then open your eyes and note down the physical and emotional feelings you discovered within your body.

Another method is to keep a stress diary. The stressful events through the day and the feelings they evoke can be recorded here. A detailed diary can be gradually completed throughout the day, or compiled in the evening by reflecting on the major events that have occurred. This allows symptoms such as headaches or backache to be correlated with stressful experiences. Over a number of weeks a pattern may emerge and situations that repeatedly cause undesirable feelings can be identified. These can then be avoided or strategies adopted to reduce the stress.

We assume that a person who has identified a problem would then wish to solve it. In practise, however, some people do not want to 'let go' of their complaint, as it is serving a useful purpose. Pain, for example, can gain the sufferer extra care and attention. This is termed 'secondary gain'. Of course it is much better, and likely to be more effective in the long run, if people can express their needs by more positive means.

Assertiveness, for example, allows people to effectively express and achieve their personal needs without detrimental effects to themselves or others. There are many such skills that can be acquired and this chapter outlines a number of them.

OVERCOMING STRESS

Gaining physical fitness requires a degree of effort, practice and perseverance, and mental 'fitness' can be achieved by similar application. There are two broad areas where new skills and techniques will achieve this goal. People can modify their stressful behaviour, while relaxation allows them to focus on attaining inner tranquillity. Many of the responses to stress have been learnt and become established habits, and these need to be replaced with new habits and attitudes so that unpleasant feelings of distress are no longer evoked. A negative attitude towards later life, as a time of worthlessness and inactivity, can be rectified by emphasizing its positive benefits and advantages. Similarly relaxation can be learnt and perfected by practice. It is not 'empty' time in which to be bored, or to brood over worries. Letting go of stressful thoughts and emotions transcends the strain of daily life by fostering inner contentment and peace of mind.

Some of the techniques to overcome stress are listed in Table 5.3. The two broad groups each consist of a number of different skills. It may be beneficial for some people to choose one technique from each category as they are complementary and achieve different results. Selecting the most appropriate method also depends on the problem that requires attention. If a sounder sleep is desired then mastering mental relaxation would be beneficial, while for the relief of muscular tension and pain massage is preferable. A technique is more likely to be effective if a person chooses it him- or herself.

You will notice that unnatural means, such as drugs, are not included in Table 5.3, and before going on to explain what these natural techniques entail, it is worth taking a look at how 'quick relief' substances actually affect us. Many people rely on alcohol, cigarettes and sedatives to relieve anxiety and tension. Any benefit is temporary and the undesirable feelings of distress soon return when the effects of these drugs have

TABLE 5.3 Techniques to overcome stress

Changing behaviour

Assertiveness training;
Organizing priorities;
Relationships;
Thought stopping;
Positive thinking;
Coping skills training;
Self-talk.

Relaxation

Autogenics;
Biofeedback;
Hypnosis;
Yoga and meditation;
Relaxation exercises.

worn off. This is frequently accompanied by a lowering of self-esteem, as people realize their vulnerability to these artificial substances, and their inability to take control of their own lives. Often, more drugs are taken in a vicious cycle that leads to dependency and addiction. Hopes of a quick, simple solution from drugs are false and misleading. In addition they have a detrimental effect on health. Smoking causes heart disease and cancer, while those who drink excessive amounts of alcohol may suffer damage to many organs of the body. Tranquillizers are addictive and abruptly stopping them after prolonged use can cause unpleasant withdrawal reactions. They therefore not only delay the resolution of problems, but themselves create new and unnecessary complications. It is preferable that natural methods, and not artificial chemicals or drugs, are used to resolve difficulties and relieve tension.

Fortunately there are many techniques that fulfil these requirements. A number, such as massage and warm mineral baths, have been used for centuries. Yoga and meditation can also be practised in their traditional form, or modified to suit the trends of modern western society. As our understanding of human psychology has increased, so too has the number of techniques for dealing with stress. There are a variety of techniques to suit different people and a number are explained here.

Warm Water

The beneficial effects of warm water have been known for centuries. Baths were an important part of the Roman culture and immersion in water is significant in a number of religious ceremonies. For many years mineral baths were used for their therapeutic properties, while more recently spas, jacuzies, hydrotherapy and flotation tanks have become popular. The buoyancy of water combined with its comforting, enveloping warmth, soothes joint pain and relaxes muscles. The addition of water jets and air bubbles massages the body. Bathing is an enforced break from the rushed daily routine, a time for peaceful relaxation. A warm soothing bath before going to bed at night frequently ensures a sounder, more restful sleep. The only precaution for people with health problems, particularly heart disease, is to first check with their doctor whether it is safe for them to take hot baths.

Massage

Massage is another effective physical therapy that has been practised by different cultures throughout the ages. Unfortunately its recent association with sexual favours has discouraged many people from trying this form of therapy. In the future increased professionalism and training will lead to a greater acceptance of massage as an important form of treatment. Although a person is usually undressed, the genitals are never touched. Oil is applied to the skin to reduce friction, and a treatment session usually lasts from half to one hour.

The massage begins with broad sweeping strokes over the whole back in order to relax the muscles. The masseur can then proceed to perform a variety of other strokes depending on the person's requirements. These include squeezing, kneading, clapping, rubbing or rolling the skin and muscles. There are alternatives to the traditional massage. Swedish massage aims to stimulate the body, while Japanese Shiatsu (applying pressure to acupuncture points) is believed to relieve symptoms and generally improve health.

The benefits of massage include relieving muscle tension and relaxing tight, knotted muscles. Physical relaxation slowly spreads throughout the body to produce mental tranquillity and a feeling of wellbeing. There is also a greater awareness and appreciation of caring for one's own body. In today's mechanized world it offers a unique experience of human closeness. Some of the more simple techniques can be mastered by an individual and used to help a spouse or friend. There are also many massage courses available, which can be attended alone or with a partner.

Muscle Relaxation

A frequent response to stress is to tense and tighten muscles. Although many people are unaware of these changes, they may eventually be brought to conscious attention by causing pain and limiting movement. Headache, neckache, backache and joint pain are all aggravated by muscle tension. In turn this discomfort increases the strain and anxiety that is already a problem. Muscle relaxation aims to reverse this cycle by loosening and relaxing the muscles, thereby reducing the feelings of distress. Each muscle is progressively tightened and relaxed in turn. At the completion of the exercise there is a pleasant loose and heavy feeling of relaxation, of having 'let go' of tension.

The following exercise can be read by a friend or taped and played back at another time. It should be read slowly and softly, with ... indicating a pause.

Exercise 2

The exercise takes approximately twenty minutes, so find a quiet place where you will not be disturbed. Lie comfortably with a cushion to support your head and loosen any tight clothing. Do not cross your arms or legs. Each muscle group is tensed for ten seconds (count to ten), followed by a period of relaxation of twice this duration (twenty seconds — but do not count).

Begin by slowly breathing in, while at the same time clenching your right fist and tightening the muscles in your right arm. Hold the muscles very tight for ten seconds ... now breathe out letting go of all the tension in your right hand and arm. Stop for a moment to enjoy the feeling of relaxation that is present in the arm . . . Repeat the same procedure for the left arm . . .

Now move on to tense the muscles of the head and neck. While breathing in close your eyes more tightly, clench the jaw and tighten the face, shoulder and neck muscles. Hold while counting to ten . . . then breathe out and feel the tension in these muscles melt away . . .

Focus on your chest, stomach, back and buttock muscles. Tighten them and feel their tension . . . Now let go . . . take your time . . . do not hurry . . .

Finally tense the muscles in your right leg, thigh and curl your toes tight . . . hold . . . relax . . .

Repeat on the left leg . . . Savour the heaviness of relaxation as it flows from the upper part of the body to engulf you in peaceful tranquillity . . .

You have now removed most of the tension from your body. If you are aware of any pockets of resistance that remain tense, tighten these muscles, hold . . . and then relax . . .

Lie here a little longer . . . enjoy the deepening bliss of relaxation . . . When you are ready open your eyes but continue resting. After a few minutes you will be fully alert but free of muscle tension.

To gain the full benefit from this exercise, it should be practised once or twice daily.

Biofeedback

This technique uses a machine to monitor and feed back information on the biological functioning of the body. As previously discussed, stress tenses muscles, causes the skin to become cold and clammy, increases heart rate and arouses the brain. These physiological changes are monitored by electrodes placed on the skin and converted to electrical impulses that are displayed as visual readings or sounds. The stress within the body can be 'recorded', and improvements can be measured after relaxation techniques have been taken up, because the sound signal or reading on the machine decreases as tension is reduced. For example, the benefits of muscle relaxation can be monitored by the biofeedback machine measuring muscle tension. With practice a person is able to recognize the signs of tension and overcome them without the use of the machine. Biofeedback can be beneficial in reducing high blood pressure, relaxing muscles, reducing tension and promoting sounder sleep.

Breathing

Today's sedentary lifestyle means people usually do not have to fully expand their lungs in the course of their daily activities. In addition tension and worry cause rapid shallow breathing, and in extreme cases this panting can lead to hyperventilation with feelings of being light-headed. Natural deep breathing to promote physical and spiritual wellbeing has been practised in eastern cultures for centuries. Recently many of these ideas on breathing have been borrowed and adapted to help people cope with the strains of modern western living.

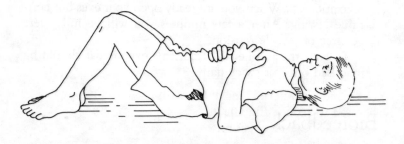

FIGURE 5.1 The posture adopted for breathing exercises.

Exercise 3

Lie comfortably on your back, loosen any tight clothing and place one hand on the chest, and the other on the stomach. Concentrate on your breathing and be aware of the hands going up while breathing in, and down while breathing out. Breathe in through your nose and out through the mouth.

Slowly take in a deep breath while counting to four. Hold for a moment and then breathe out more slowly counting to eight. Repeat this until a regular rhythm is established and then allow the counting to fade away. As the air is expelled from the lungs imagine the tension and worry leaving the body. They are carried out with the exhaled air. Quietly repeat the word 'relax' as you breathe out.

Allow more problems to flow out with each breath. Feel the clean fresh air fill every corner of the lungs.

Focus attention on the remainder of your body, as the goodness of oxygen spreads to all the muscles and organs. It restores vitality to tired parts of the body and carries away the tension, to be expelled when breathing out. Experience the pleasure of relaxed deep breathing.

This deep peaceful breathing should be continued for five to ten minutes, and performed once or twice each day. After mastering the technique in the restful lying position it can be performed on other occasions to immediately deal with stress. While sitting or standing in a queue, the frustration of these situations can be countered by starting deep, peaceful breathing.

Imagery

Thoughts and images that are conceived in the mind are known to affect bodily functions. Everyone has experienced the sensation of saliva being produced while visualizing a delicious 'mouth watering' meal. Similarly, peaceful thoughts can be used to reduce the effects of stress on the body. The imagery can be a recollection of previous pleasant experiences or it may be fictitious. Frequently the images used for relaxation are related to nature. Wind-swept beaches, picturesque mountains, forests with babbling streams are often associated with holidays and contribute to a feeling of tranquillity. It is important to visualize every detail of the scene, as this ensures it will be more realistic.

The exercise described below is only one example of an imagery technique. It is preferable for everyone to visualize their own peaceful scene. It can be written down, recorded and then replayed while sitting or lying comfortably with the eyes closed. Set aside five to ten minutes for this exercise. Begin by using a breathing or muscle relaxation technique —

being relaxed frees the mind of worries and helps a person to enter their imaginary world more easily.

Exercise 4

Imagine your favourite place ... It may be an inside place or outside place ... It may be your favourite room ... or a place where you spent your most satisfying holiday ... You may have been there only once ... or visited it many times ... Wherever it is ... it is your place ...

Now picture yourself there ... Are you sitting or standing? ... Are there other people or animals with you? ... Look around ... Take in every detail ... the colours ... the smells ... the feeling of the air against your face ... Explore it ... Know it well ...

Experience again that comfortable feeling ... Feel it engulf your whole body ... your neck ... shoulders ... back ... and stomach ... Take your time ... let the sensation stay with you ... Take a last look around ... say goodbye knowing that you can return to your special place whenever you wish ...

It is also possible to use imagery to cope with stressful situations and relationships. Even when the circumstances themselves cannot be altered, this technique can reduce the anxiety they evoke within an individual.

Exercise 5

Close your eyes. Breath slowly and deeply ... Say 'relax' as you breathe out ... Feel the muscles loosen ...

Look around for your problems and worries. They may be thoughts you wish to possess no longer ... ideas that make you feel uneasy ... people who have made your life miserable ... unhappy events ... or circumstances that are unpleasant. Some may be hidden so search your mind to find them all ... Gather them together ...

Having collected these thoughts, look for a place where they can be disposed of forever. In the distance, on top of a hill, you see a colourful hot air balloon ... It is a difficult journey but you make steady progress and gradually approach your destination ... Struggle up the hill with your load until you reach the top . . . As you come closer the balloon is seen more clearly. It is beautiful and contains all the colours of the rainbow . . .

Examine individually each item you have been carrying . . . each problem . . . each worry . . . each hassle. Know it well before loading it into the basket of the balloon . . . Say goodbye as you part with each one, as this is the last time you will see them . . . Cover the top of the basket and lock it securely so nothing can ever escape . . . Move back in preparation for the launch. Count from ten to zero, and then there is liftoff . . .

Watch the balloon climb above the trees . . . It is carrying all your problems and worries away . . . The clouds part to allow the balloon through . . . It drifts higher and higher . . . All that you wanted to be rid of is carried further and further away . . . It is now barely visible . . . Wait until it can no longer be seen . . . Feel the relief of being free.

Imagery can also be used to improve self-esteem and encourage acceptance of the new roles in later life. A person can visualize themselves as confident, energetic and leading an active healthy lifestyle. Dreaming of holidays, setting new goals and planning new ventures are all ideas that can germinate in a free-thinking mind and grow to fruition with subsequent planning and action. Solutions to difficulties can be envisaged and practised mentally in preparation for meeting and overcoming obstacles. Recalling previous successes and glories not only reinforces self-worth, but provides an example for overcoming present difficulties. The power of imagery can be an important resource for those who wish to successfully enjoy later life free of worries and tension.

Hypnosis

Hypnosis is a useful technique to induce relaxation. It produces an alteration in conscious awareness which is best described as a trance-like state, being between fully awake and in a deep sleep. The feeling is similar to day-dreaming and the calm experienced just before falling asleep. Hypnosis is a technique that should be practised by a qualified hypnotherapist, although some people may eventually master self-hypnosis and use it to help themselves control and understand aspects of their own lives.

The hypnotic state is induced by the hypnotherapist, who encourages subjects to focus their attention and eliminate all distractions. This is often done by the therapist repeating calmly and continuously instructions that invite a change in the conscious state. Suggestions that the subjects are feeling sleepy and drowsy, or to close their eyes as the eyelids become heavier and heavier are commonly used themes. Alternatively, they can fix their attention on a pendulum, bright light or object in the room. Uninterrupted gazing and concentrating on these objects leads a person into a hypnotic trance. Individuals cannot be hypnotized against their will and are aware of what is occurring during a treatment session. They remain in control and can awaken from this hypnotic trance if they desire.

Hypnosis has many interesting effects. These range from a reduction of pain, to 'age regression' which involves reliving experiences from a younger age, including childhood. Even bodily functions such as heart rate and sweating can be affected. An important benefit of hypnosis is its ability to induce inner calm. Often, people are able to 'access' past experiences that cannot be recalled while fully conscious. Unresolved problems can be dealt with in this way, but only by an experienced and qualified therapist. Post-hypnotic suggestions are instructions the therapist will make while the subject is still in a trance, but she or he will perform them when fully conscious. Positive post-hypnotic suggestions can improve sleep, bolster self-esteem and help a person cope with difficulties. Hypnosis offers many benefits for an older person. These include reducing anxiety, altering behaviour to improve the response to stress, and pain relief.

Autogenics

Autogenic training is a form of self-hypnosis which is achieved by people responding to their own instructions. These self-suggested thoughts aim to exert an influence on bodily functions such as circulation, muscle tension, heart rate and breathing. As previously explained, stress results in a number of physiological changes including elevation of blood pressure, palpitations, indigestion, neckache and cold, clammy hands. Autogenic training reverses these changes and returns the body to a stable, relaxed equilibrium. Biofeedback is frequently used in conjunction with autogenics to monitor its effectiveness in reducing these reactions to stress.

People can choose the sensations they wish to alter and then formulate a phrase which expresses their aspirations. This should be silently repeated while concentrating on that part of the body. The most commonly used auto-suggestion aims to influence the feelings experienced in an arm (or leg). Silently repeating the phrase 'my arm is feeling heavy and warm' while focusing on the arm will, with practice, lead to improved circulation and relaxation of the muscles in that limb. Having mastered and gained control over this part of the body, a person can then move to alter heart rate, breathing and digestion, and regain peace of mind if these have been adversely affected by stress.

Before starting autogenic training it is advisable to have a medical check-up, as vital organs such as the heart are going to be affected. Some people also notice side effects in the initial stages of autogenic training. These are usually transitory, but if they persist it is important to seek a therapist's advice. The side effects (also termed 'autogenic discharges') can include unexpected physical reactions such as muscle aching and twitching, caused by the release into the muscles of tension that has been suppressed for many years. Emotional reactions such as sadness and crying can result from the exercise, removing some of the person's psychological defences to reveal underlying unresolved conflicts.

Exercise 6

The following are auto-suggestive phrases which are applicable to various parts of the body:

Limbs — My arm is heavy ... My leg is heavy ... My arms and legs are heavy.
My arm is warm ... My leg is warm ... My arms and legs are warm.
My arms and legs are heavy and warm.
Heart — My heartbeat is calm and regular.
Breathing — My breathing is deep and even.

Solar plexus — My stomach is warm and pleasant.
Head — My forehead is cool and relaxed.

Autogenic exercises are most beneficial if they are performed
for short periods (one to two minutes) but frequently (five to
eight times) throughout the day. Sitting in a comfortable
chair or lying are the positions recommended for these exercises. Each instruction is repeated four times. The method
suggested in *The Relaxation and Stress Reduction Workbook* (by
Martha Davis, Elizabeth Eshelman and Matthew McKay) is
a progressive twelve-week programme involving the inclusion
of different parts of the body on a weekly basis as each stage
is mastered. The first week concentrates on heavy feelings in
the limbs, and progresses to encompass warmth in the limbs,
regulation of heartbeat and breathing, solar plexus (digestion)
and finally the head. The person is in a state of 'passive
concentration'; aware of what is occurring but not trying to
influence it. At the end of the exercise there is a feeling of
being both relaxed and alert.

Meditation, Yoga and Tai-chi

The philosophy of these ancient eastern practices is based on
the belief that there is a harmonious unity between the body,
mind and spirit. An improvement in physical and mental
health can be achieved by learning these techniques from a
qualified teacher and practising them regularly.

Meditation aims for serenity and peace of mind by directing
a person to focus their attention on inner thoughts and feelings. The mind can be disciplined to achieve this by concentrating intently on only one thing. The focus of thought
can be breathing, or a part of the body (commonly the centre
of the forehead, termed 'the third eye'). Images, scenes and
objects are other subjects that can be used as the central
theme for focusing thoughts. *Transcendental meditation* involves concentrating on a single word or 'mantra' which is
repeated many times. Meditation frees the mind of unpleasant
thoughts and if it wanders can easily be brought back to concentrate on the subject. Intrusive thoughts that are concerned
with everyday problems are excluded, allowing the mind to
be clear and still.

Prayers are interpreted by some to be a form of meditation. The ritual forces individuals to break their daily routine, to relax and concentrate on one thing, in this case religious prayer. It can impart an aura that transcends everyday life and offers a universal perspective to personal problems.

Yoga emphasizes the close relationship between the mind and body. It is regarded as both physical and mental exercising. The various poses increase awareness of one's own body and improves flexibility. This physical freedom is believed to free the mind of stress and engender an inner peace. For older people it is advisable to be instructed in yoga by a qualified teacher, who can assess the most appropriate exercises with which to begin, and modify them as greater flexibility is achieved through practise.

Tai chi is an ancient Chinese art that combines meditation with movement. The exercises are graceful and flowing, requiring concentration to follow the precise sequence of actions. Again, the slow, relaxed pace of movement brings with it inner contentment and greater satisfaction from life.

Thought-stopping

Thought-stopping involves taking control and stopping thoughts that provoke anxiety. For example, people who ruminate about their health are preoccupied with every ache and pain, and their wellbeing would improve if they were free of this obsession.

The first step is to define the upsetting thoughts. Next concentrate on each one for a fixed period of time, usually one to three minutes. When this time has passed shout 'STOP!' and immediately clear those thoughts from the mind. Fortunately, with practice this can be done internally, without verbalizing 'stop'! If initially it is difficult to control these thoughts, activities can be undertaken that distract attention from them. Alternatively pleasant thoughts can be substituted to displace those that are not wanted.

Self-talk

Self-talk is the internal thought process that expresses a person's own point of view about themselves and the world around them. This in turn affects attitude and feelings. Positive self-talk enhances self-esteem and personal endeavours are more likely to be successful. Examples of positive self-talk include: '*I can overcome this problem*', and '*I am a worthwhile person*'.

The interpretation, or self-talk related to an event, is often the cause of anxiety, rather than the event itself. Much of a person's negative self-talk is based on irrational ideas. Ten such misconceptions are listed in Table 5.4. Albert Ellis, who proposed this concept, believed that these false beliefs result in unnecessary feelings of distress. He suggested that the strain an individual experienced would be reduced by closely examining and questioning the evidence for these beliefs. Frequently the conclusion would be that the premises were false and based an misconceptions or distortions.

Formulating objective rational beliefs and substituting these for the false misconceptions results in positive self-talk and an optimistic approach to life. For example, the first irrational idea listed in Table 5.4 suggests that people expect to be approved of by everyone they meet. It is impossible for this to always occur, and a more rational approach would be to recognize that many, but not all people, will like you. Those who do not are entitled to their opinion, but this should not result

TABLE 5.4 Irrational ideas

1. It is imperative that I am loved and approved of by everyone I meet.
2. To be a worthwhile person, I must be competent and perfect in all my endeavours.
3. Any misfortune is punishment for being bad and wicked.
4. It is disastrous when things don't turn out the way I would like them to.
5. Unhappiness is due to external factors which are beyond my control and therefore cannot be altered.
6. I cannot stop myself worrying about things that are uncertain or potentially dangerous.
7. It is easier to postpone than tackle difficult issues and obligations.
8. I need to rely on someone stronger than myself.
9. Present difficulties are caused by past experiences and therefore cannot be changed.
10. Other people's problems and worries should be adopted as my own even if they cause similar feelings of distress.

in feelings of disappointment and negative self-talk. The myths of later life that portray older people as useless, inflexible and feeble-minded fall into this category, and reflect society's prejudices towards older people. For this to change older people themselves must dispel these false myths from their own minds.

Stress Innoculation

This method of coping with stress involves planning how to deal with a problem so that when it is encountered feelings of anxiety are not provoked. The first stage is to define the stressful events. The person can then devise an alternative and relaxed response that will allow the same problem to be successfully dealt with on the next occasion. This may involve repeating a phrase that reinforces thoughts on how to best overcome the problem, or simply learning to relax through breathing and muscle relaxation. These strategies are then rehearsed and implemented when next the problem is confronted. For example, if visiting a sick friend in hospital creates unpleasant feelings, these can be overcome by imagining a visit to the hospital and initiating relaxation by deep breathing immediately this distress is experienced. With practice, the visitor will automatically feel more at ease on future occasions. This can be enhanced by repeating a phrase such as 'I can see this visit is making my friend happy and I can cope with staying longer'. When the situation is no longer a source of stress, self-congratulations are indicated!

Positive Thinking

Many prophecies about the future are self-fulfilling, and it is therefore imperative to have a positive outlook on life. If people perceive later life pessimistically as a time of boredom and inactivity it is unlikely they will become motivated to embark on projects that will result in a different outcome. Problems can also be redefined so that the positive aspects are emphasized. The grief following the death of a spouse can be viewed as an expression of love for that person and should therefore not be suppressed by false bravado. Living and enjoying the present, viewing later life as an important part of the life cycle and an opportunity to embark on new ventures, is preferable to dwelling on the past or being apprehensive about the future.

Assertiveness Training

Assertiveness ensures that individuals safeguard and achieve their personal rights while still respecting the rights of others. It is a preferable approach and usually more successful than being either aggressive or passive. People who are too hostile and aggressive antagonize others, while those who are passive and withdrawn are unlikely to succeed in achieving their aims. Assertive behaviour involves being direct, calm but firm in communicating one's rights and desires. This results in less stress and improved, more open relationships. As we saw in Chapter 2, it is particularly important for carers of an ill relative or friend not to neglect their own needs. Being assertive allows these people to explain their reasons for taking a break, while ensuring that the needs of the ill person are not neglected. In the long term this is preferable to becoming over-burdened to a point where they can no longer cope and resent their role as caregiver.

Assertive behaviour can be learnt. Begin by recalling and evaluating situations that need to be changed. Imagine the scene but then substitute behaviour that is more assertive. This can be reinforced by writing down the imagined dialogue and rehearsing it many times until the behaviour becomes familiar. Practising in front of a mirror helps to develop body language skills that are a vital part of being assertive. Assertive behaviour reduces stress; a person is likely to communicate more effectively and succeed in achieving what he or she wants from life. There are now many courses that teach assertiveness.

Problem-solving

Problems are unavoidable, with success and happiness being determined by how they are approached and solved. The critical first requirement is to clearly define the problem. This is followed by 'brainstorming' for different ideas and solutions. All possibilities are listed without considering whether they

are practical or the best option. When the full range of alternatives has been exhausted, each should be evaluated. The best
solution can then be decided. In later life, for example, it is
not uncommon to feel disappointed and restless after retirement. This problem may be due to an excessive amount of
free time. Having defined the problem, list all activities which
can be undertaken to combat these negative feelings. Family
and friends can all contribute their ideas, but in the end it
is the individual who must make the decision on which
activity or activities will be taken up.

Time Management

Older people can enjoy a more fulfilling, balanced life by
allowing adequate time for a broad range of activities. These
should include work, recreation, exercise and relaxation. In
later life there is a wide variation in the need for time
management. Some people may be over-committed and
always rushed, while others have an abundance of spare time

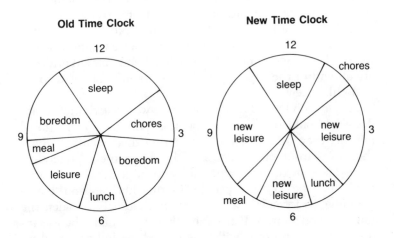

FIGURE 5.2 Time management time clocks.

and become bored. Both these difficulties can be overcome by careful preparation and planning.

In order to make the best possible use of the time available a person should first set the priorities and goals which she or he wishes to achieve. The present allocation of time should be examined and decisions made regarding how it can be used more efficiently. A daily schedule can be formulated by dividing the day into half or one hour units, and allocating different activities according to the priorities that had been set.

Recreation

Throughout life there must be time for play. Due to the pressures of work and financial commitments this aspect of life can be neglected, so that people entering later life may have forgotten how to enjoy themselves. Recreational activities are a source of fun and happiness, complementing relaxation to improve the quality of life. They prevent the build-up of stress by distracting attention from problems and displacing thoughts that provoke anxiety.

The range of possible pastimes is enormous. Included are sports, hobbies, clubs and intellectual pursuits. Most commonly it is the activities that were started in youth or middle age that are continued throughout life. In order to facilitate a smooth transition to later life, a variety of activities could be tried before retirement. This does not preclude initiating something new or unconventional. Higher education, learning to play an instrument, bush walking and veteran athletics are all within the capacity of those who are motivated to try something new.

People who have difficulty deciding which activities to undertake should recall those hobbies, sports and recreational pursuits they were interested in during their youth. Perhaps there was insufficient time to fully enjoy them previously. Later life provides the opportunity to fulfil these past ambitions. Talking to other people, visiting libraries and 'brainstorming' to formulate a list of alternatives will broaden the range of possibilities. If the initiative is not taken by the individual, then nothing will change, and the full potential for an enjoyable life will not be achieved.

Relationships

Friendships with other people protect against the adverse effects of stress. Problems can be discussed and solutions found with support from family and friends. There is even evidence to suggest that those who have a supportive relationship, such as marriage, are likely to live longer. During a crisis relatives and friends can offer both practical and emotional support, keeping morale high with understanding, encouragement and praise.

Taking the initiative oneself is the best way to establish new relationships. For these to continue it is important to maintain communication. Listen to other people's opinions and attitudes. Acknowledge their feelings and points of view, even if they are different. An accepting easy-going attitude allows friendships to flourish.

Love and romance can develop from a close friendship, adding an extra dimension to the relationship. Sexual intimacy not only gives pleasure, but is also very relaxing. It reinforces a person's self-worth by emphasizing that he or she is physically desirable.

Another important source of companionship for some people is their pet. It has long been recognized that pets have a calming effect on their owners. An animal's unconditional devotion is important to many people who may otherwise be lonely. Walking a dog, for example, also provides an opportunity to meet and chat with neighbours and other people who may have similar interests.

Nutrition

There is a close association between stress and nutrition. Not only does an inadequate diet make an individual more vulnerable to the effects of stress, but stress itself is often the cause of nutritional problems. As a reaction to pressures and worries some people lose their appetite and so do not consume an adequate amount of food. A stressed person will often not take the time to prepare meals. At the other extreme there are those who react by over-eating and gain weight. Despite this their nutrition can be inadequate, as the food consumed is often poor quality 'fast foods' which are high in kilojoules but deficient in vital nutrients. Stress also increases the demand for certain vitamins, particularly the B group. This compounds the problem of obtaining sufficient nutrients during times of stress.

It is important to eat a balanced and varied diet which is low in fat, salt and sugar but contains natural produce such as fruit, vegetables and whole grain cereals together with some protein rich food (meat and fish). Meals are a time for relaxation, with the food being eaten in a calm unhurried manner. It can also be used as an opportunity for social interaction with friends and family. Those who eat a healthy balanced diet are more likely to successfully cope with the stresses of life.

Exercise

Regular physical exercise results in good health, a relaxed positive attitude to life and a feeling of being in control. Fit people cope better with stress and suffer less tension, anxiety and depression. One possible explanation for this is related to the natural hormones, adrenalin and endorphines, that are released in response to stress. Adrenalin, which causes many of the unwanted reactions to stress, is consumed during exercise, allowing the body to return to its natural resting state. Complementing these changes are the second group of hormones called endorphines. These are released into the brain, resulting in relaxation and a feeling of wellbeing. A number of physiological benefits are also associated with regular exercise and reverse the effects of stress. Heart rate and blood pressure are lowered, while tight, tense muscles become loose and relaxed after exercising. Exercise is also invigorating, with fit people suffering less tiredness and fatigue.

Special consideration should be given to the factors that ensure an exercise is relaxing and enjoyable. Frequently people push their bodies beyond comfortable limits and although this may still be beneficial to physical fitness, it detracts from the pleasure that can be derived from such activities. The discomfort endured can also prompt them to stop exercising. Moderation is important; the exercise should be vigorous enough to be physically beneficial but should remain within sensible limits. Competition also diminishes the relaxing influence of exercising. Competitive sports can still be played, of course, but it is important to differentiate between these and exercises which are relaxing.

Activities can be incorporated into the daily routine so that they do not become an inconvenient burden. Pleasant surroundings such as a park or beach, perhaps combined with listening to music, will also enhance the enjoyment of exercise.

CONCLUSION

All the techniques described above rely on the individual taking responsibility for her or his own health, and initiating ways of dealing with stress and reducing anxiety. Invariably there will be setbacks and problems before the techniques are fully mastered. It is important not to be discouraged but to accept it as a normal part of gaining a new skill. The aquisition of these new habits usually does not occur all at once, but progresses in stages. Setting short term goals, and reinforcing success by rewarding progress, are two ways which will encourage success. If no improvement is noticed or the problems seem insurmountable, then it is wise to seek the advice of a doctor or psychologist. Age need not be a barrier to reducing the unpleasant effects of stress.

6 DRUGS

> . . . they do not heal, but only relieve
> suffering temporarily, exchanging one disease
> for another.
>
> Mary Baker Eddy

It is often assumed that 'the drug problem' is restricted to young people who use illicit drugs such as heroin and marijuana. In fact it is the legal drugs, namely alcohol and tobacco, that cause more health problems. This misconception arises from society's approval of certain substances as 'acceptable', when in fact there is little distinction between the adverse effects of those that are legal and those that are not. Figures released during 'The Drug Offensive' reveal that of the 21 000 deaths attributed to drug use, the vast majority are due to cigarettes and alcohol. Cigarettes accounted for over 71 per cent of deaths, alcohol 26 per cent and opiates only 1 per cent (Figure 6.1). The detrimental effects of smoking and alcohol usually take many years to develop, and therefore manifest themselves as diseases in later life.

Another less obvious drug problem is related to prescribed medication. The increasing prevalence of illness with advancing age, combined with the expectation that almost all of these ailments can be remedied by medication, has resulted in many older people consuming excessive amounts of medication. This frequently results in drug interactions and unwanted adverse effects, and some of these can be serious.

The main drug problems facing those in later life are related to cigarettes, alcohol and prescribed medication. The degree to which each of these is harmful varies. While all smoking is detrimental to health, alcohol in moderation is acceptable, and medication if used correctly can be beneficial. Theoretically all drug related illnesses and deaths can be prevented by discouraging people from smoking, limiting the amount of alcohol consumed and by using medication correctly. This chapter will deal with the problems of drug use in later life, how they can be prevented and what steps can be taken if the misuse of drugs is already a problem.

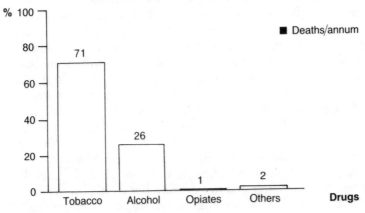

FIGURE 6.1 Drug related deaths in Australia (1987).

SMOKING

Almost 18 000 Australians die each year from smoking related diseases. Smoking is known to contribute to both heart disease and cancer, the two leading causes of death. In fact one third of all cancer deaths are due to smoking. Viewing this from a different perspective, it has been calculated that smoking one cigarette shortens the smoker's life by seven minutes, while a person who smokes twenty cigarettes each day will lose five years of his or her life. Even passive smoking, inhaling air polluted with other people's side-smoke, has been linked to lung cancer in adults and chest infections in children. Despite the overwhelming evidence warning people about the dangers of smoking, 20–30 per cent of Australians over fifty years of age continue this unhealthy habit. The good news is that the number is gradually decreasing, and that many people who continue to smoke would like to stop. Most importantly, it is still beneficial for people in later life to stop, even if they have smoked for many years. It is not too late.

Understanding the reasons that compel people to continue smoking can help them break the habit and quit. One of the main urges to continue is their dependence on the drug nicotine contained in cigarettes. Like all physical addictions there is a strong drive to keep on using the drug rather than suffer the distressing effects of withdrawal. Smoking is often used as a means of relieving tension. Other people rely on it for a 'boost' and to aid concentration. These effects are the result of smoking triggering chemical changes within the body. It causes the release of endorphines which relax the smoker and impart a feeling of wellbeing. It also stimulates the release of adrenalin which alerts the brain and improves concentration. The other main attraction of smoking is related to behavioural and social factors. The whole ritual of 'lighting up' is often initiated by certain activities such as talking on the phone, driving and drinking coffee or alcohol. A smoker often finds it impossible to separate her or his behaviour on these occasions from smoking. These so-called 'advantages' of smoking must be weighed against the dangers to health a person risks by continuing to smoke.

The Hazards of Smoking

The hazards of smoking can be best understood by examining the different components of the smoke inhaled and their effects on the body. The drug *nicotine* plays a critical role in establishing a person's dependence on cigarettes. Nicotine acts as a stimulant, causing an increase in heart rate and blood pressure. These changes, combined with a rise in the level of blood fats and a narrowing of the arteries caused by smoking, contribute to heart disease. The platelets in the blood also become more sticky, causing the blood to clot more easily. If a clot develop in the arteries to the heart the person suffers a heart attack, with smokers also having a greater risk of sudden death from heart disease. In the bronchial tubes and lungs, coughing is suppressed by nicotine which paralyses the tiny protective hair-like cilia which line the respiratory tract. Damaging particles are not cleared, and this leads to chest infections and a number of lung diseases. Nicotine is also believed to accelerate skin ageing; it reduces the blood flow to the skin, depriving it of nourishment.

Carbon monoxide, the same poisonous gas that is discharged from a car's exhaust, is also present in cigarette smoke. It binds to the red blood cells and prevents oxygen from attaching. Consequently oxygen, which is essential to good health and proper functioning of the body, reaches the muscles and organs in reduced amounts. This decreases physical fitness and may also contribute to heart disease.

Most people are familiar with the brown stains on smokers' fingers and teeth caused by cigarettes — this is due to *tar*. Tar consists of many different chemicals, some of which are known to cause cancer of the lung, bladder, mouth and throat.

The final main group of harmful substances inhaled in cigarette smoke are the *irritant particles*. These are deposited on the walls of the respiratory tract, triggering a cough (commonly called a 'smokers' cough'). Continued exposure leads to bronchitis. If the particles go on to reach deep inside the lungs, they destroy the air sacs, causing scarring and emphysema. The end result of repeatedly exposing the body to the drugs and pollutants in cigarette smoke is the development of a number of diseases. These are listed below:

Heart
- hypertension;
- stroke;
- heart attack, sudden death from heart disease, angina;
- peripheral vascular disease (hardening of the arteries to the legs causing pain and gangrene if untreated);
- aortic aneurysm (weakening, ballooning and rupture of the main artery in the body).

Lungs
- lung cancer;
- bronchitis;
- emphysema;
- respiratory infections;
- cancer of the mouth and throat.

Gastro-intestinal system
- cancer of the oesophagus (gullet), stomach and pancreas;
- peptic ulcer.

Reproductive System
- cancer of the bladder and cervix;
- irregular periods;
- earlier menopause (two years);
- impotence (reduced blood supply).

Others
- osteoporosis;
- skin ageing;
- reduced fitness.

The Benefits of Quitting

People in later life often feel that they are too old to stop a lifelong habit of smoking, and may consider that 'the damage has already been done'. Recent research has revealed that this is incorrect, and that improvements in health can be demonstrated even in people over sixty-five who stop smoking. Within one year the risk of developing heart disease is halved, and after ten years is reduced to that of a non-smoker. The risk of developing lung cancer can also be significantly decreased, although this can take a longer time to achieve. With one quarter of life still remaining, there is ample time to enjoy the benefits of improved health. All the diseases listed above can be prevented by not smoking, with the rewards for ex-smokers ranging from a healthier heart and lungs, to an improved sex life. In addition, a person simply feels better and more healthy now that their body is rid of the chemicals and drugs contained in cigarettes. No longer a slave to nicotine, these individuals have gained greater control over their lives, and this improves self-confidence. They often look more attractive and their skin seems younger. Fingers and teeth are no longer tarnished by nicotine stains, and the stale smell of tobacco is gone. Smell and taste improve, so enjoyable activities such as eating are enhanced. The money saved by not buying increasingly expensive cigarettes can be used for more worthwhile purposes. Even family and friends benefit as they are no longer being exposed to the harmful effects of side-smoke. The strength and determination of an older person quitting can also serve as an example to younger people.

How to Quit

Careful consideration of the damage to health caused by smoking, combined with the many advantages of becoming a non-smoker, will persuade most people to stop. A number are successful on their first attempt and require no special advice or support. Suffering a smoking related illness can also be an important incentive to stop immediately. Others may not triumph until their third or fourth try, but as this is not unusual a person should not be discouraged if their initial efforts are unsuccessful. The benefits gained from quitting are just as worthwhile whether it is the first or fifth attempt.

After deciding to quit smoking, the next step is to set a definite date for this to occur. Special occasions such as birthdays or holidays are often useful choices. Drawing up a contract with a friend will increase motivation and improve the chances of success. Informing close family and friends not only gains their support, but also enables them to understand the reason for any changes in behaviour that may occur during the initial stages of withdrawal.

The urge to smoke is largely due to the person being physically addicted to nicotine. Smokers maintain a constant level of this drug in their bloodstream by smoking an adequate number of cigarettes. When the level of nicotine starts to fall they experience a craving for tobacco. Within seven seconds of smoking a cigarette the blood level of nicotine starts to rise again. As with all drugs of addiction, ceasing the drug causes symptoms of withdrawal. These include feelings of irritability, anxiety and poor concentration. Headaches are common, as are mouth ulcers and digestive complaints. The craving for tobacco can be very intense. These unpleasant effects of withdrawal are strongest during the first few days after stopping, and have usually subsided after two weeks. Knowing that withdrawal is normal and will settle after a short time enables a person to persevere until this difficult period has passed.

The undesirable effects of withdrawal can be reduced by tapering off the dose of nicotine. In practice this involves gradually reducing to a minimum the number of cigarettes smoked and the amount of nicotine inhaled. There are numerous ways this can be achieved, but they have in common the effect of breaking established smoking habits or making it an unpleasant activity. A person can begin by smoking only half a cigarette, inhaling less deeply and restricting smoking to only certain situations, for example never smoking indoors. Alternatively, rationing cigarettes and smoking only those that are 'essential', will often significantly reduce the number smoked. The urge to have a cigarette can be controlled by delaying 'lighting up' for ten minutes. Regularly changing brands and also smoking those that are not the person's favourite, makes it a less enjoyable activity. Many people smoke automatically. Placing rubber bands around packets and buying single packets instead of cartons increases a smoker's awareness of his or her habit, so that it can be altered.

Another consideration when quitting is to overcome the psychological dependence on cigarettes with its associated social rituals. This involves learning new habits and alternative strategies to replace the satisfaction previously obtained from smoking. Cigarettes are often used by smokers as a prop in their social interactions with other people. As mentioned, they also relieve some of the unpleasant feelings associated with stress and improve concentration. In order to master this aspect of smoking it may be necessary to record in a diary when each cigarette is smoked and the activity or feelings with which it is associated. In this way the factors that trigger the desire for a cigarette can be recognized, and changes made to overcome them. The habit of smoking after a meal, for example, can be anticipated and thwarted by planning an activity such as a walk immediately after finishing the meal. Social gatherings are frequently a trap. It is advisable never to accept cigarettes when they are offered, and on social occasions to associate with non-smokers. People who continue smoking frequently feel threatened by a person who is in the process of stopping, and may try to sabotage her or his efforts. Alcohol is often a trigger for smoking and should be avoided. If there is a need for oral gratification to replace the satisfaction obtained from cigarettes, then chewing gum or sipping water and fruit juices can be substituted. Some people are fidgety and miss the ritual of handling and lighting up cigarettes. Fiddling with coins and worry beads, or taking up hobbies such as drawing and knitting, which occupy the hands, will satisfy this need. As each obstacle is overcome and the fight against smoking is won, it is important for people to congratulate and reward themselves for their success.

It is essential to stop smoking completely. Simply cutting down or changing to a brand with a lower tar and nicotine content is fraught with difficulties. Studies have shown that when a person chooses to do this there is often a change in the way they smoke. Inhaling more deeply in order to obtain the same amount of nicotine to satisfy their body's craving is common. As a result more of the harmful substances such as tar and carbon monoxide are also absorbed. Because the tar and nicotine content is lower there is a misconception that these cigarettes are safe and more can be smoked. With continued smoking, even if only one or two per day, the potential also exists for this to increase if the person is subjected to unexpected stress. Zero is the only safe number of cigarettes to smoke.

TABLE 6.1 Tips for quitting

- Be confident, positive and optimistic about stopping;
- Decide to quit after suffering a smoking related illness;
- Enlist the support of family and friends;
- Stop completely and don't just cut down or change brands;
- Dispose of smoking paraphernalia (ashtrays, lighters etc);
- Craving for cigarettes is normal and will subside;
- Do not try 'just one' cigarette as a test;
- Anticipate difficulties and plan how they can be overcome;
- Avoid situations that trigger smoking;
- Change the daily routine so that smoking is excluded, for example exercise regularly; (it is impossible to smoke while swimming!)
- Weight gain is no excuse to delay quitting; the risks to health from smoking are far greater than those of being overweight;
- Weight gain is not inevitable and can be prevented by healthy eating and regular exercise;
- Indulge in a reward with the money saved from not buying cigarettes;
- Self-congratulations are in order for each successful day a person does not smoke;
- Failure is not uncommon so do not be discouraged; instead try again.

Other Methods of Quitting

There are a number of other choices available to smokers who wish to quit. Hypnosis and acupuncture can be very useful. 'Rapid smoking' is an approach which emphasises the unpleasant effects of smoking. It involves rapidly inhaling cigarette smoke every six seconds. After approximately fifteen minutes an excessive amount of nicotine has been absorbed and the smoker starts to feel nauseated and may vomit. This drastic procedure has proved beneficial in helping those in later life to stop smoking. It should be performed under medical supervision and used with caution in people with heart and lung complaints.

The intense withdrawal reaction experienced by some people when they stop smoking can be cushioned by using a chewing gum that contains nicotine ('Nicorette'). Initially, it can be used as a substitute for cigarettes, and whenever there is an urge to smoke another piece of gum is chewed. The nicotine is absorbed from the mouth, a process which is slower than smoking in raising the nicotine level of the blood, and therefore for some people not as satisfying. Nicotine gum cannot be chewed like normal chewing gum. The technique is summarized as follows:

- There are two doses of gum, 2 mg and 4 mg, with 2 mg gum being equivalent to half a cigarette.
- The gum should be chewed slowly over twenty to thirty minutes.
- After ten to fifteen chews rest the gum between the cheek and teeth until more is required.
  - Too vigorous chewing causes nausea, a sore tongue, indigestion and hiccups;
  - Insufficient chewing does not satisfy the craving for nicotine.
- Gradually reduce and then stop using the gum.
- Three months is the longest time the gum should be used.
- People with heart disease and ulcers should consult their doctor before taking nicotine gum.

Finally there are specially designed programmes that guide a person through the difficult first few weeks after quitting.

They educate the smoker about the harmful effects of cigarettes and help them to understand their reasons for smoking. In addition there is a great deal of support offered to those who find it difficult to quit. These programmes are organized by the Anti-Cancer Councils in most states and are particularly beneficial for people who have tried unsuccessfully to stop smoking.

ALCOHOL

The widespread consumption of alcohol as a socially acceptable beverage belies the fact that it is a drug. There is no doubting its ability to produce a relaxed feeling of wellbeing which many people enjoy. In this way alcohol serves as a 'lubricant' for social interaction. But the potential for causing damage is always present, depending on the amount consumed. Its main effect on the body is sedation, which is achieved by depressing the nervous system. Small amounts are harmless but as more is consumed the number of problems rises and diseases can develop. If extremely large amounts of alcohol are ingested alcoholic poisoning can occur. Using alcohol to relieve tension or solve problems is not advised; this can easily lead to abuse.

Alcohol drunk in excess over a long period of time will lead to physical addiction and symptoms of withdrawal when it is stopped. In addition, tolerance develops so that more alcohol must be consumed to achieve the same effects. Eventually it becomes the most important part of that person's life, assuming a higher priority than family, work and health. It can lead to family conflicts, job loss and ill health. The National Health and Medical Research Council has recommended safe levels of alcohol consumption. These are outlined below:

One 'standard' drink contains 8–10 grams of alcohol, which equals —
200 ml of beer;
90 ml of wine;
60 ml of fortified wine (port, sherry), or
30 ml of a spirit (whiskey, brandy, liqueurs).

Light consumption is up to two drinks for women; and up to four drinks for men.

Medium consumption is two to four drinks for women; and four to six drinks for men. Light consumption is unlikely to cause problems, but with medium consumption there is a risk of developing alcohol related problems, including damage to important organs.

Heavy consumption is more than four drinks for women, and more than six drinks for men. This is where drinking becomes hazardous, often resulting in physical and mental deterioration, as well as social problems. If the intake is more than twelve drinks per day then damage is inevitable.

Alcohol and Disease

Alcohol affects almost every organ of the body. An excessive intake is associated with many illnesses, which lead to unnecessary suffering and a reduced lifespan. A number of problems are listed below. If the excessive consumption of alcohol is not prolonged, then a number of these diseases can be reversed. Unfortunately this is often not the case, and many conditions such as cirrhosis of the liver and nerve damage (peripheral neuropathy) are irreversible once they have developed. When alcohol is combined with smoking the risk of mouth, throat and gullet cancer significantly increases. On a brighter note, there is evidence to suggest that a small amount of alcohol (one to two glasses a day) may be beneficial in reducing the incidence of heart disease by favourably altering the blood fats. Listed below are the ways alcohol affects the body:

Nervous System
- deterioration in memory and intellect;
- peripheral neuropathy (numbness and pins-and-needles in the limbs);
- Wernicke-Korsakoff syndrome (disorientation, memory loss and blackouts);
- epilepsy;
- cerebellar ataxia (loss of co-ordination and unsteadiness);
- dementia.

Gastro Intestinal
- liver-hepatitis and cirrhosis;
- gastritis and ulcers;
- pancreatitis;
- diarrhoea.

Heart
- cardiomyopathy (disease of heart muscle);
- high blood pressure.

Muscle
- myopathy (weakening of the muscles).

Blood
- anaemia.

Nutrition
- vitamin deficiencies (especially Thiamin-B1),
- poor dietary intake/malnutrition.

Psychological
- depression;
- anxiety;
- suicide.

Sex
- impotence.

Social
- breakdown of relationships with family and friends;
- economic hardship;
- car accidents.

Alcohol and Later Life

There is a general reduction in alcohol intake with age. However the altered metabolism and increased sensitivity of organs such as the brain to drugs, causes alcohol to have a greater effect on people in later life. A reduction in alcohol consumption is therefore desirable. Although people suffer from alcoholism in later life, this is less common, and is in part due to many alcoholics having died prematurely. In addition, concerns about health encourages many older people to examine their lifestyle and modify practices such as smoking and drinking, which are known to be detrimental to health.

Alcoholism

Alcoholism in older people is more prevalent in women than men. The majority (two thirds) of older alcoholics are chronic long-term drinkers, having consumed excessive amounts of alcohol over many years. For the remainder it is a relatively recent problem which has developed in response to the stresses of later life. If difficulties such as bereavement, boredom and loneliness cannot be coped with satisfactorily, a person may turn to alcohol to relieve the unpleasant feelings. Unfortunately this creates a vicious cycle which prevents the resolution of these problems.

The first and most important step towards treatment of alcoholism is awareness of the problem. Many people find this very difficult, and strongly deny they have a problem. Recognising all the dangers of continued drinking and the advantages of stopping may motivate some to abstain or at least modify their consumption of alcohol.

It is common for alcoholics to suffer withdrawal symptoms such as tremors, hallucinations and sweating when alcohol is no longer consumed. In these circumstances it is wise to be under the care of a doctor, who may feel it is necessary to prescribe vitamins and occasionally other medication. Informing relatives and friends of a person's intention to stop drinking will enlist their co-operation and support, ensuring a greater chance of success.

Examining the factors that led to the alcoholism and endeavouring to overcome them will help prevent people from slipping back into old habits. If boredom and loneliness were the cause, then new activities, voluntary or part-time work and joining a social club are practical solutions. Professional counselling on personal problems is also beneficial. Alcoholics Anonymous is a self-help group that encourages people to take responsibility for their own actions, and will also help the spouses of alcoholics. Attending Alcoholics Anonymous meetings has been shown to be particularly successful for those who have started drinking excessively in later life as a response to stress; age should not be a barrier to overcoming alcoholism.

Caffeine

Caffeine is a mild stimulant that is widely consumed in coffee, tea, chocolate and cola drinks. Coffee contains the highest amount of caffeine, approximately twice as much as tea. The caffeine content of other drinks is listed in Table 6.2. The stimulating effect of caffeine increases the heart and breathing rate, as well as causing mental arousal. Excessive amounts of caffeine can result in insomnia, palpitations and feelings of anxiety. It is also addictive and when ceased a person may suffer withdrawal symptoms such as headaches and tiredness. To prevent these problems from developing, it is advisable to limit the amount of caffeine to 300 mg each day, which is equivalent to three to four cups of instant coffee.

Recent reports linking caffeine with heart disease and various cancers have been proven incorrect. Its association with heart disease, for example, is more likely due to the sedentary and smoking habits of coffee drinkers, rather than the direct effect of caffeine. Caffeine is, however, known to aggravate osteoporosis (thinning of bones).

TABLE 6.2 Caffeine content of food and beverages (mg)

Coffee (1 cup)	
Percolated	100–150*
Drip filter	100–120*
Instant	80–100
Decaffeinated	2–4
Tea (1 cup)	10–90*
Hot chocolate (1 cup)	50–70
Cola drinks — 370 ml can	45
Chocolate bar, 30 g	20

* Varies depending on strength of the brew and type of beans and tea leaves.

MEDICATION

From ancient times humans have sought to cure their ailments with medication. Modern medicine has gone far beyond the plants and herbs once used; indeed, many people now expect that drugs will cure almost any ailment, that there is 'a pill for every ill'. This attitude often results in pressure on both the doctor and the patient; it is expected that medication will always be prescribed, even when it may not be the best alternative. Although drugs are invaluable in curing some conditions, the majority improve a person's quality of life by alleviating and controlling the symptoms of disease. Many ailments, such as arthritis and heart disease, are chronic and may be present for years. In order to be free of unwanted symptoms, medications may need to be taken for long periods of time. With advancing age there is an increased incidence of these chronic diseases and therefore more tablets are taken. Research has revealed that at least 80 per cent of people over sixty-five years of age take some form of medication, either prescribed or purchased over the counter. Although people in this age group represent less than 10 per cent of the population in Australia, they consume 25 per cent of drugs prescribed.

Medication can be both beneficial and problematic. The physiological changes of ageing which alter the body's ability to handle drugs, together with the greater number of drugs taken, contribute to more adverse reactions being experienced. The undesirable effects of drugs are two to three times more prevalent in older people. There is a wide variation in the types of problems suffered, ranging from minor inconveniences to severe reactions requiring admission to hospital. In one survey, a quarter of elderly people admitted to hospital were found to be suffering from complaints related to their drugs.

It is often difficult to recognize adverse drug reactions. They can be non-specific, mimicking both age and disease. Feelings of weakness, tiredness, dizziness and nausea are examples. These may be accepted as a normal part of ageing, and may not even be mentioned to the prescribing doctor. When they are mentioned, they may not be recognized as being due to medication. It is not uncommon in such circumstances for a doctor to prescribe yet another tablet to relieve the additional symptoms; the original problem remains and may in fact be aggravated by the extra medication. Frequently people themselves do not wish to stop their tablets for fear that the original problem will return. This is often further compounded by patients who expect to receive a prescription for each new complaint. It is clear that both patients and their medical attendants need to be educated about the appropriate use of drugs for the treatment of illness in later life.

Problems are also encountered if psychological and social difficulties are inappropriately treated with medication. Bereavement, social isolation and financial worries are experienced by a number of people in later life. Although they present to their doctor with a variety of physical complaints a thorough examination will often reveal that no illness is present. Rather than taking medication to relieve physical symptoms, it is more sensible for people to seek a solution for their personal difficulties, which are the real cause of distress. Obtaining support from family, friends or community organizations, attending a professional counsellor to resolve grief or a financial adviser for money matters, are more appropriate and result in permanent solutions.

The Action of Drugs and Ageing

The increased susceptibility of those in later life to the adverse effects of drugs can be partly explained by the biological changes associated with ageing. There is an alteration in the way drugs are handled, which modifies their effect on bodily functions. Although a number of general guidelines exist, there is great variability not only amongst individuals but also between different drugs. Unfortunately, much of the research into drugs is carried out on young and middle-aged subjects, so that the results and recommended dosages are not always applicable to older people. The altered action of drugs due to age is best understood by examining the different processes they undergo as they pass through the body. Drugs are first absorbed, then distributed around the body so that they can exert their actions, and finally excreted.

Although there are a number of changes that theoretically could affect drug *absorption*, this is not necessarily the case in practice. However the *distribution* of drugs throughout the body is altered as the result of less body water and a relative increase in body fat. Less body water means that water soluble drugs will become more concentrated and may even cause toxic reactions. On the other hand, drugs such as tranquillizers, which can accumulate in the extra fat, usually do not reach dangerously high levels in the blood. However, as they are slowly released from the body fat, these drugs can have an unacceptably prolonged period of action. In the case of tranquillizers this can result in drowsiness and a 'hang-over' effect.

Having exerted their influence most drugs are then *metabolized* (broken down) by the liver before leaving the body. The decrease in blood supply to the liver, together with a reduction in its size, are both the result of ageing. These changes slow the metabolism of certain drugs, particularly tranquillizers, and as a result they remain in the body for a longer period of time. This does not occur with all drugs, but the explanation is complex and is beyond the scope of this book. Finally, drugs are *excreted* by the kidneys. Kidney function is also known to slowly decline with advancing years and consequently causes drugs to reach higher than normal levels in the bloodstream.

The body's sensitivity to different drugs is altered by age. A full range of all the possibilities is complicated, but it is important to note that the brain becomes more sensitive to tranquillizers, which can result in excessive drowsiness. The normal response to many other drugs is also impaired and this results in significant adverse effects being experienced. Dizziness, confusion and urinary incontinence are infrequent but well recognized serious consequences which reflect these difficulties.

All the above problems are compounded by the high number of medications taken by those in later life. These drugs compete and interact, resulting in more frequent and severe reactions. The multiple prescribing of drugs is termed *polypharmacy*, and is often the result of a person suffering from a number of diseases. Consulting different doctors for each complaint can result in drugs being prescribed without consideration of their overall effect on those already taken for other conditions.

Serious illnesses usually require drugs to control them, but many others can be alleviated without medication. Physiotherapy for arthritic pain and relaxation to relieve tension are examples. In addition to the biological changes of ageing which cause problems with prescribed medication, human factors are also important.

Compliance and Acceptance of Medication

There are many problems that can occur between the time a doctor writes a prescription and the patient actually takes the medication. If a misunderstanding results in an insufficient amount of the drug being taken, the treatment will be ineffective, while toxic reactions are likely if the dose is excessive. Compliance as a medical term is used to describe a patient's ability to follow a doctor's instructions. Unfortunately it implies submission and even blame on the part of the patient if the medication is incorrectly taken. Ensuring that tablets are correctly taken is really a shared responsibility between the manufacturer of the drug, the prescribing doctor, the pharmacist who dispenses the medication, and finally the patient who takes it. Acceptance is preferable, since it indicates that a person is willing to take the medication, knowing its benefits, side effects and the correct dose.

It is estimated that between 25–60 per cent of prescribed medications are taken incorrectly, and this is generally not due to ageing or the result of forgetfulness. The most frequent reason is the underuse of prescribed medication, often because unacceptable drug reactions are experienced. Excessive and inappropriate taking of tablets also occurs. This can be the result of hoarding old tablets, and even swapping or taking other people's medication!

A number of these difficulties can be reduced by keeping the number of tablets to a minimum, and the dose simple. Labelling and instructions must be clear, with expiry dates and warning labels clearly visible. To date no special consideration has been given to people with poor vision and those who cannot read English. The manufacturer also has a responsibility to ensure that the size and taste of their tablets are acceptable for an older person to handle and swallow. Packaging should be easy to manage, unlike a number of the present 'child proof' containers which people with arthritis may have difficulty opening.

Doctors remain the major source of information, and it is important that they clearly communicate all the necessary facts to their patients. This should include an explanation of the problem, the reason for medication, how it should be taken and the expected duration of treatment. If side effects are likely this should be explained and the patient advised what to do if they occur. If these points are not discussed, a person should not feel too inhibited to ask for this information. Extra care must be taken to ensure that if an individual attends a number of different doctors, they all communicate with each other to minimize duplication and interaction of drugs. The pharmacist is another valuable resource person who can provide additional advice related to taking medication.

A small number of people are at a high risk of having problems with their drugs. These include individuals with poor vision and hearing, who require special consideration in order to understand instructions. People suffering from dementia need either a family member or a visiting nurse to administer and monitor their drugs. Finally, those who are alone and neglected by their families often are depressed, and do not care how their medication is taken. Greater consideration and care to the special problems of those in later life are important in the manufacture, prescribing, and consumption of medication. This will reduce the incidence of adverse effects and prevent unnecessary illness and suffering.

Over-the-counter Medication

Most people do not consider the pharmaceutical items they purchase without a prescription to be medication. One estimate is that 83 per cent of people in later life take over-the-counter preparations, with antacids, laxatives and tablets to relieve pain being the most common. Although it is desirable that individuals demonstrate their independence by trying to relieve minor complaints, these medications are not without problems and should be regarded as drugs. Some 'cold and flu' remedies elevate blood pressure, while the humble aspirin can cause stomach ulcers and bleeding. More commonly difficulties arise when these medications interact with prescribed drugs. An example of this is the decreased effectiveness of certain antibiotics if they are taken with antacids. It is therefore advisable to check with either the pharmacist or doctor before taking over-the-counter medication. Alcohol also significantly interferes with prescribed drugs, although it is purchased over a different counter!

Common Drug Related Problems

Although drugs have the potential to cause problems in people of any age, those in later life have more frequent adverse drug reactions. In order to maintain a true perspective of this problem, it is important to emphasize that in the majority of cases the prescribed medication is both necessary and beneficial. Most people never suffer side effects, but when problems do arise it is essential that they are recognized and action is taken to rectify the situation. If a person suspects that their medication is causing a problem, he or she should discuss it with a doctor. Simply ceasing the medication may cause a deterioration in health. However, if the complaint is ignored by the doctor or the explanation offered is unsatisfactory, then a second opinion should be sought.

A major cause of concern is the consumption of 'nerve tablets' in later life. Statistics reveal that older people take 55 per cent of all such tablets prescribed, and that they are taken more often by women than men. The most commonly used drugs are the benzodiazepines, of which Valium, Serepax and Mogadon are examples. Frequently sedatives are prescribed to settle the symptoms of anxiety associated with a crisis. In certain circumstances they may be indicated, but if taken for longer than two weeks addiction can develop. These sedatives are often continued unnecessarily for many years after the original problem has been resolved. Another reason for the over consumption of tranquillizers and sleeping tablets is in the treatment of sleeplessness. With increasing age it is normal for sleep to be of shorter duration and to be interrupted by periods of waking. Sleeping tablets are therefore not needed once a person is aware that this is the normal pattern of sleep in later life.

Tolerance and addiction can also become problems for people who take tranquillizers over a long period of time. As tolerance develops larger doses are required to achieve the same effects. Addiction to these drugs causes a withdrawal reaction when they are ceased; feelings of tension, aches and pains, insomnia and dizziness are common. Instead of coping with these symptoms the drug is usually continued, often indefinitely. There is no doubt that many people should consider stopping their 'nerve tablets' but this should be done very slowly and under medical supervision.

A number of common side effects are listed below. They range from minor annoyances such as a dry mouth, to potentially devastating disabilities. If any of these symptoms occur, a doctor should be consulted.

TABLE 6.3 Side effects of commonly used drugs

Prescribed medication

Fluid tablets (diuretics)

- dry mouth, dehydration;
- blood pressure falls with changes in posture;
- confusion;
- urinary incontinence;
- biochemical imbalance — gout, raised blood sugar, body depleted of potassium;
- interference in social activities (frequent visits to the toilet).

Heart and blood pressure tablets

Digoxin

- nausea, vomiting and diarrhoea;
- irregular heart beat (can result in dizziness and falls);
- confusion

Beta-blockers

- slow pulse;
- heart failure;
- asthma;
- reduced circulation to the limbs;
- reduced exercise tolerance;
- postural fall in blood pressure;

- falls;
- confusion.

Blood pressure tablets
- postural fall in blood pressure;
- tiredness.

Nerve tablets — sedatives and sleeping tablets

Minor tranquillizers (Benzodiazepines)
- addiction and withdrawal reactions;
- drowsiness, dizziness, feelings of a 'hangover';
- confusion;
- incontinence (sleeping tablets may cause incontinence at night);
- falls.

Major tranquillizers
- symptoms similar to Parkinson's Disease;
- postural drop in blood pressure;
- confusion;
- falls.

Anti-depressants
- dry mouth;
- constipation and urinary retention;
- postural fall in blood pressure;
- heart problems;
- confusion.

Arthritis tablets (non-steroidal anti-inflammatory drugs)

- indigestion, bleeding from the bowel;
- kidney damage;
- fluid retention;
- skin rash.

Antibiotics

Co-trimoxizol
- kidney damage.

Over the counter medication

Pain relieving tablets

Paracetamol
- liver and kidney damage if taken in excess.

Aspirin
- indigestion, bleeding from the bowel;
- kidney damage;
- 'thins' the blood, prolongs bleeding.

Codeine
- constipation.

Laxatives

- damage to the bowel;
- interferes with the absorption of food, especially some vitamins.

Cold and flu remedies

These are often a combination of a number of different drugs:

Paracetamol, Aspirin, Codeine,
See above.

Ephidrine, Pseudoephedrine
- elevates blood pressure;
- aggravates heart problems.

Antihistamines
- drowsiness, tiredness;
- dizziness.

Antacids

- interfere with other drugs, especially antibiotics (tetracyclene);
- disturbance in bowel function, constipation and diarrhoea;
- alteration of body's biochemical balance, e.g. sodium (salt) elevates blood pressure, and calcium raises calcium blood levels.

Vitamins

Excessive amounts of vitamins can produce side effects for example:

Vitamin A
- toxic effects (damage to hair, skin and bone).

Vitamin B6
- flushing, dizziness.

Vitamin D
- high levels of calcium (vomiting, headaches).

Vitamin C
- kidney stones.

Preventing Problems with Medication

In theory all problems related to medication can be prevented. To achieve this ideal many changes are needed, but some are beyond the immediate control of an individual. These relate to the negative stereotype of later life, with illness and discomfort being accepted by many people as a normal part of ageing. Doctors and other health professionals often reflect this stereotype, and accept as part of ageing complaints that are in fact due to the side effects of drugs. In addition, greater emphasis on the benefits of disease prevention in general, as well as the prevention and early detection of adverse drug reactions, is much needed. Drug companies also have to consider the needs of the elderly. The size, shape, colour and packaging of medication are all issues that need to be addressed. If people in later life assert their rights as important consumers of health services, then together they may achieve many of these changes.

In order to minimize the risk of drug reactions a fundamental change in attitude towards medication may be required. Put simply, many conditions can be remedied without medication. Blood pressure, for instance, can be lowered by reducing weight and decreasing the amount of salt eaten in the diet. Pain in certain situations can be relieved by biofeedback, acupuncture and applying electrical nerve stimulation to the skin. The majority of personal and emotional difficulties are best resolved without drugs, by counselling, relaxation and learning new coping skills.

Certain problems with medication can be prevented by improving the exchange of information between doctor and patient. Before attending their doctor people should decide which problems they wish to discuss so that none are overlooked at the time of the consultation. Noting these down may be helpful. Also list all current medication and any side effects that are suspected. During the consultation do not hesitate to become involved by enquiring into the nature of the problem and the various treatment options available. Ask if there are any alternative treatments that are as effective but do not involve drugs. Should medication be required it is important to clearly understand its benefits, if side effects are common, and what to do if they occur. Practical details must also be explained. These should include how often tablets are to be taken and whether there are any special instructions, such as taking them with food. If people are un-happy with some aspect of the treatment they should voice their objection. For example, if it is necessary to take a tablet at midday, but a person is never at home at this time, it is preferable to explain this, rather than simply omitting that dose. A point often overlooked is to enquire how long the medication should be continued. Writing this information down in a special drug booklet for future reference will prevent any misunderstanding, and can be used to inform other health professionals, such as pharmacists and specialists, of the current medications.

A crucial part of a medical consultation is the relationship that develops between a person and her or his doctor. If the doctor views later life negatively or is unwilling to provide all the information that is sought, the patient as a consumer should consider changing doctors. Health is an important part of later life and often involves on-going treatment. Deciding on the best alternatives for treatment should be by mutual agreement after a two way discussion between the doctor and patient. Greater involvement and taking responsibility for one's own health is likely to lead to fewer problems from all forms of drugs. Below are listed some of the questions to ask your doctor or pharmacist*:

Questions to ask your doctor
* Are there any alternatives to medication?
* If I need a medicine, what is its name?
* What is it for? What will it do? How long do I have to take it?
* How do I take it?
* What if I miss a dose?
* What should I do if I experience any side effects?
* Do I need a repeat?

---

* From: 'Before you take it . . . talk about it! Produced by the Australian Consumer's Association.

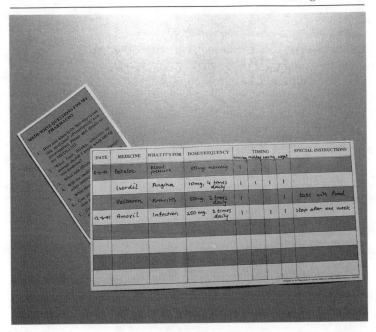

DATE	MEDICINE	WHAT IT'S FOR	DOSE/FREQUENCY	TIMING morning	midday	evening	night	SPECIAL INSTRUCTIONS
6-6-91	Betaloc	Blood pressure	50mg. morning	1				
	Isordil	Angina	10mg, 4 times daily	1	1	1	1	
	Voltaren	Arthritis	50mg, 2 times daily	1				take with food
12-6-91	Amoxil	Infection	250 mg. 3 times daily	1		1	1	stop after one week

FIGURE 6.2 A sample medication chart.

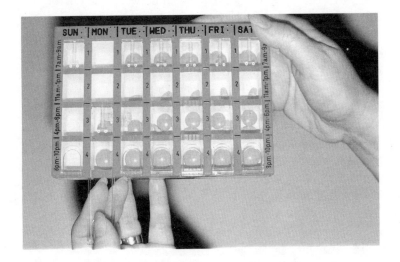

FIGURE 6.3 A drug dispenser.

Questions to ask your pharmacist
* Can I take this medicine with the other medicines I am taking?
* Is the container easy to open?
* Will you explain the label to me?
* Will you put what the medication is for on the label? (e.g. heart tablets, water tablets)
* How should I store the medicine?

7 PREVENTION OF COMMON HEALTH PROBLEMS

'An ounce of prevention is worth a pound of cure.'

The aim of prevention is to reduce the risk of illness, avoid disability and delay death. The emphasis moves from the treatment of diseases by a doctor, to the person accepting responsibility for her or his own health and wellbeing. This self-care includes eating a balanced diet, engaging in regular exercise and being able to cope with stress. These are all practices that are within an individual's control.

People are living almost twenty years longer than their ancestors at the turn of the century and this is largely due to improved hygiene and better living conditions, preventive measures that are today accepted as normal. The challenge for the future is to extend life expectancy even more by preventing the chronic diseases that are prevalent in later life. An equally important challenge is to lengthen older people's period of good health, so that they remain active and independent.

PREVENTION AND RISK FACTORS

Many of the diseases common in later life, including heart disease, stroke and cancer, are preventable. The recent decline in the number of deaths due to heart disease and stroke cannot be attributed to improvements in treatment alone. Greater community awareness and acceptance of a number of preventive measures is also believed to have played an important role.

The chronic diseases prevalent today do not have an obvious single cause. There are a number of contributing factors, termed *risk factors*. In the case of heart disease, for example, these factors include smoking, high cholesterol and high blood pressure. Eliminating or modifying these risk factors will prevent, or at the very least delay, the development of heart disease.

Although certain ailments often first appear in later life the disease process itself starts much earlier. The fatty deposits that cause heart disease are known to be present even in twenty-year-olds. It is therefore important to institute preventive health measures as early as possible. This of course raises the question of whether prevention is necessary, or even applicable, to people past middle age.

PREVENTION IN LATER LIFE

My second marriage was to a woman eight years younger who wanted to have another child. I calculated that when our daughter turned twenty-one I would be seventy-four. From the time my wife became pregnant I worked on improving my health. I have stopped smoking, I exercise regularly and take care with the foods I eat. Now at sixty-eight I feel better and fitter than I did fifteen years ago. I am confident we will all celebrate her twenty-first birthday together.

David (68)

A healthy lifestyle can prevent illness in later life. The disease process does not alter with age, so the same risk factors apply at all stages of life. As noted in Chapter 6, if people aged sixty stop smoking they will benefit from less heart disease, the risk decreasing by 50 per cent after one year. Strokes have been linked to high blood pressure. If this condition is treated effectively in later life the incidence of stroke will also be reduced. Exercise has also been shown to lower the death rate even in people aged seventy to eight-five years. In short, it is wrong to think that unhealthy practices are no longer relevant or harmful in later life.

What cannot be disputed is that a number of factors relevant in youth and middle age may not apply to the same degree in later life. For example, the relationship between high cholesterol and heart disease is less significant in older people. Despite this, a connection does exist and those at risk of developing heart disease are well advised to eat a healthy diet. Based on present information, however, aggressive treatment of high cholesterol with medication in older people remains contentious.

Preventative measures for the elderly have been neglected because it is often assumed that disease already exists. Advice to alter lifestyle at this 'late' stage is often considered pointless and equivalent to 'closing the barn door after the horse has bolted'. This argument is best answered by understanding how diseases develop. Atherosclerosis or hardening of the arteries is a good example here. Poor lifestyle habits, such as smoking and eating an unhealthy diet, accelerate the accumulation of fatty tissue (plaque) along the walls of arteries, causing them to become narrow. At a certain point this significantly reduces the supply of blood reaching the heart and the person will begin to notice symptoms of heart disease. Most people in later life have already accumulated a certain amount of fatty plaque in their arteries, but the amount may still not be sufficient to cause problems. Modifying the risk factors, such as stopping smoking, will slow the disease process. The postponement of symptoms, due to an improved lifestyle, is still possible in later life, enabling the individual to remain healthy for longer.

The aim of prevention is to postpone illness to a short period of time immediately prior to death. Figure 7.1 demonstrates this idea. The development of illness in a smoker (a) begins early in life. The breathlessness due to emphysema is experienced at a relatively young age, followed by a heart attack and stroke, also at a young age. The person is unlikely to completely recover from these serious ailments leading to chronic ill health, dependency and frequently institutional care. Eventually, after years of suffering, lung cancer develops and is the final cause of death. An alternative scenario (b) is to delay the development of these diseases by leading a healthy life which always includes not smoking. As a result the person is unlikely to suffer from emphysema or become ill at a young age. He or she will remain independent and in good health until in the twilight of life a heart attack and stroke in quick succession lead to death.

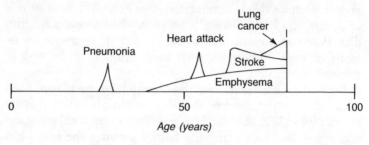

Prototypic lingering chronic illness

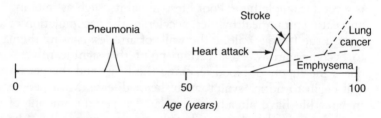

Effects of the postponement of chronic disease

FIGURE 7.1 Effects of the postponement of chronic disease.

PREVENTION IN PRACTICE

Prevention can operate in a number of ways. These range from suggesting healthy lifestyle habits that slow the development of diseases, to preventing disability once a disease has become established. Regular exercise, healthy eating and avoiding harmful drugs such as cigarettes and alcohol are all measures that prevent disease. The greatest benefit is obtained if these are started as early as possible.

In addition to physical illness, the prevention of emotional problems is highly desirable. Adverse stress and anxiety as the result of difficulties with retirement, housing or finance can often be avoided by adequate preparation and planning. A preventive health plan should include physical, emotional and social factors, since they are all involved in maintaining good health.

Complications in illness can be prevented and treatment is more successful if diseases are detected early. A regular 'check-up' is advisable — it will often reveal unrecognized problems. Tests can also be useful in diagnosing disease before symptoms appear. Many screening tests are available. The smear test for women is an essential routine test for women of all ages. Mammography (X-ray of the breasts) as a screening procedure for breast cancer is also gaining support and its implementation in Australia is currently being assessed.

Once a disease has become established the emphasis shifts to minimize any adverse effects on normal living. Arthritis is common in later life, but even those with quite severe arthritis can remain self-sufficient and independent with the help of various aids and modifications to their environment.

To summarize, there are three levels of prevention. A healthy lifestyle is the most effective way to avoid illness. If this is not successful then early detection of the problem will improve the chance of a cure. Finally, when a disease becomes established, preventing dependence and disability should become the next goal.

DISEASES OF THE HEART AND BLOOD VESSELS

Diseases of the heart and blood vessels are the most common cause of death in Australia, claiming almost half the number of people who die each year. Included in this group are heart attacks, high blood pressure and strokes. There has been a welcome decrease of approximately 45 per cent in the incidence of deaths due to heart disease and stroke over the last twenty to thirty years. This improvement is believed to be due to advances both in the treatment of these conditions and, more importantly, healthy living. In the absence of disease the heart and blood vessels continue to function well in older people. Although a risk factor, ageing alone is not the main cause for the increased incidence of these ailments in later life, which are due to the damaging effects of *atherosclerosis*.

Atherosclerosis

Atherosclerosis is the accumulation of yellow, fatty deposits along the walls of arteries, which weakens and narrows these blood vessels. As a result the supply of blood to the tissues nourished by that artery is reduced, while the weakened wall of large vessels is liable to rupture. The surface of the artery damaged by atherosclerosis is irregular and rough, similar to the accumulation of rust in corroded pipes. Small clots may develop on the roughened surface of these fatty plaques, causing a complete blockage and the sudden interruption of the blood supply. Tissues supplied by that artery are starved of oxygen and die.

Atherosclerosis starts at a young age and progresses silently until, in middle and later life, sufficient damage has occurred to cause symptoms of disease. High blood pressure, smoking and high blood cholesterol levels accelerate this process. Avoiding these risk factors will prevent the development of atherosclerosis. Recent exciting research has revealed that reducing cholesterol levels can *reverse* this process, with noticeable improvements being reported after two years. This may have important implications for those in later life who have usually accumulated a considerable number of fatty plaques.

Atherosclerosis affects almost all arteries of the body and manifests itself as a number of separate diseases. Arteries to the heart, brain, and legs are particularly vulnerable, resulting in some of the more common diseases. It is worth considering each of these areas in more detail.

Heart Disease

In the development of heart disease, the coronary (heart) arteries become narrow due to atherosclerosis. This reduces the amount of blood reaching the heart, depriving it of vital oxygen and nutrients. During exercise, when the heart has to work harder, there is insufficient oxygen for the heart's needs, causing chest pains which subside after a period of rest. These chest pains are termed *angina*. The heart does not sustain any permanent damage as the result of angina, but the pain should not be ignored because it reflects underlying heart disease. Treatment of angina may reduce the possibility of a heart attack as well as relieving these chest pains.

A person suffers a *heart attack* (coronary, myocardial infarct) when the coronary artery that supplies the heart becomes completely blocked by a small blood clot suddenly developing on the surface of one of these fatty plaques. The section of heart muscle that is deprived of oxygen dies and in time a scar forms in its place. Unfortunately, often it is only after a heart attack that people first examine the way of life that has contributed to ill health.

Prevention of Heart Disease

Heart disease is common in developed countries such as Australia and the United States, suggesting that it is related to an affluent lifestyle. A number of factors increase the possibility of a person developing heart disease. These factors account for two thirds of the cases of heart disease, suggesting that other, as yet unrecognized factors, may also be involved.

There has been some controversy regarding the relevance of these risk factors to people in later life. It has been argued that those at greatest risk die in young and middle age, making the risk factors less relevant to older people who are 'survivors'. Unfortunately much of the original research linking heart disease and lifestyle excluded older people, but recent studies have started to clarify this problem. Based on the available evidence it is generally agreed that people of all ages will improve their health by modifying the risk factors known to cause heart disease. The benefits may not be as dramatic as those gained if the preventive measures had been introduced at a younger age, nevertheless, for most the effort will be worthwhile.

The National Heart Foundation has formulated a list of risk factors that contribute to heart disease, and many of these can be modified by changes in lifestyle:

Major risk factors
- Family history
- Male sex   Non-modifiable
- Age

- Smoking
- High blood pressure
- Raised blood fats   Modifiable
- Obesity

Other factors
- Lack of exercise
- Diabetes
- Excessive alcohol
- Stress

When factors interact their adverse effects are compounded. Therefore if more than one risk factor is present the possibility of heart disease is significantly increased; the combination of two to three risk factors results in a proportionally greater increase in the likelihood of a heart attack.

Non-Modifiable Risk Factors

Increasing *age* is associated with a higher incidence of heart disease, and obviously this cannot be altered. Men in youth and middle age have a greater risk of developing heart disease, but in old age both sexes are equally at risk. The most important non-modifiable risk factor is a *family history* of heart disease. If a close relative (mother, father, brother or sister) suffered a heart attack or angina, there is an increased risk that other members of the family will develop similar problems. This should not be interpreted as a prediction of gloom, but should act as an incentive to modify other risk factors.

Smoking

Smoking is the most lethal risk factor — a smoker's chances of developing heart disease are doubled. In addition, smokers have a greater chance of sudden death due to fatal irregular heart beats. Smoking causes heart disease in a number of ways. It damages the walls of arteries which accelerates atherosclerosis, and the inhaled poisonous carbon monoxide displaces oxygen in the blood which reduces the supply of oxygen to the tissues. Nicotine also has an important effect as it increases the heart rate and raises blood pressure.

The risk of heart disease is halved after not smoking for one year, and is the same as a non-smoker after ten years. Smokers are strongly advised to quit, and the benefits of improved health can be enjoyed after a relatively short period of time.

High Blood Pressure

High blood pressure places an extra strain on the heart which must work harder to pump the blood against this higher pressure. It also damages the arteries, accelerating atherosclerosis. Lowering the blood pressure prevents these problems and reduces the risk of heart disease. Checking blood pressure is a simple procedure that should be performed at least twice each year.

Raised Blood Fats

There is no question that lowering blood cholesterol and to a lesser extent triglyceride levels reduces the risk of heart disease. It has been shown that a 1 per cent reduction in blood cholesterol lessens the risk of heart disease by 2 per cent. However, the association between blood cholesterol and heart disease is less pronounced in later life.

Blood cholesterol can be routinely checked every five years. It is estimated that half the population of Australia have a cholesterol reading above the acceptable level of 5.5 mmol/l. Readers should turn back to pages 95–9 for an extensive discussion of cholesterol, and how to lower it.

Obesity

Obesity is a widespread problem; it is estimated that half the people over fifty-five are overweight. Carrying extra weight is an added strain for the heart, and contributes to high blood pressures, diabetes and raised levels of fats in the blood. The distribution of weight is also thought to be important. People who carry the excess weight around their waist (apple shape) are at greater risk than those who gain weight on their hips (pear shape). Maintenance of a normal body weight through healthy eating and moderate exercise reduces the risk of heart disease.

Lack of Exercise

Sedentary people are more likely to develop heart disease than those who are active. Exercise reduces the risk by improving the circulation to the heart and ensuring that it functions more efficiently. In addition exercise prevents obesity, lowers blood pressure and favourably alters the level of blood fats. Prior to undertaking exercise it is advisable to undergo a full medical check-up. The rewards of improved fitness are many and those wishing to start an exercise programme should read Chapter 3, where it is dealt with in greater detail.

Diabetes

The elevated levels of sugar in the bloodstream of diabetics contributes to the development of heart disease. Diabetics who maintain good control of their diabetes by eating a balanced diet will reduce their risk of developing this serious complication. Blood cholesterol and triglyceride levels are often also elevated due to diabetes; it is therefore important that these are regularly checked. Fortunately the treatment for diabetes and the prevention of heart disease overlap, with the emphasis being on healthy eating and regular, moderate exercise.

Alcohol

There is some evidence that a small amount of alcohol (one to two glasses per day) reduces the risk of heart disease. Amounts greater than this frequently have adverse effects by increasing the blood pressure and raising the level of fats, particularly triglycerides, in the blood. Large amounts of alcohol can directly damage the heart.

Stress

Stress contributes to the development of heart disease. Anxiety is known to raise the blood pressure and pulse rate as well as cause irregular heart beats. Other risk factors such as smoking, poor eating habits and lack of exercise are also associated with stress, because people under pressure frequently do not have the time or motivation to improve their way of life.

As previously discussed (p. 121), certain behaviour is more likely to result in stress and heart disease. People who are typically competitive, impatient and achievement-orientated put themselves at greater risk. Relaxation techniques, discussed in Chapter 5, should be used to overcome this problem.

Preventing Complications

In the event of suffering a heart attack, a person should go to a hospital as quickly as possible. Recent advances in treatment enable the extent of the heart damage to be minimized by administering drugs to dissolve the clot blocking the artery to the heart. Dangerous heart irregularities can also be promptly and effectively treated in hospital.

Preventing Further Heart Attacks

> After my heart attack and bypass surgery I became very depressed and felt my days were numbered. I was keen to stay healthy and followed the heart specialist's advice. I have stopped smoking, lost weight, (although not as much weight as I would like) and walk almost every day. In a strange way I feel lucky that I have been given a second chance, as I now feel healthier than before the heart attack and enjoy my life more.
>
> Bill (61)

After a heart attack people frequently feel vulnerable to further ill health and choose to embrace a healthy lifestyle. They are motivated to correct the risk factors previously discussed including obesity, smoking, high blood pressure and cholesterol levels. Advice on exercise is also generally sought.

A number of medications have also been shown to be beneficial. *Aspirin* 'thins' the blood, preventing the formation of blood clots which block the heart arteries and cause further heart attacks. In addition another group of drugs, called *Beta blockers*, are effective in reducing heart problems in the first two years after a heart attack. Both these medications should be taken *only* if prescribed by a doctor, as they can have undesirable side effects.

Increasingly *heart surgery* is being performed, and a number of specific blockages in the arteries to the heart are best treated in this way. It is important to emphasize that this does not apply to everyone with heart disease and careful testing is performed before selecting those who will benefit. In addition surgery can relieve angina and reduce or even eliminate the need for medication. Modern technology now also offers choices other than surgery. Narrow arteries are widened by inserting a small balloon, which is inflated. Alternatively, the fatty plaque can be removed by a special cutting instrument. More recently lasers have been used, but require further evaluation before becoming generally available. Although there is a certain risk involved, many people are now able to enjoy a more active, independent life as a result of these surgical procedures.

Stroke

A stroke occurs when an artery in the brain becomes blocked or ruptures, cutting off the supply of oxygen and nutrients. That area of the brain dies and the corresponding part of the body it controls cannot function. For example, damage to the part of the brain controlling movement in the leg will lead to difficulty in walking. As is the case with heart disease, atherosclerosis is the underlying disease process that causes strokes. A narrowed artery in the brain can become completely blocked due to a blood clot forming on the surface of a fatty plaque. Clots can also form in the heart or arteries of the neck and travel to the brain where they become lodged, obstructing the flow of blood. The most serious damage occurs when a weakened blood vessel bursts, causing bleeding into the brain. Fortunately this is the least common cause of a stroke.

Although the majority of people survive a stroke many will continue to suffer a disability that interferes with their previous way of life. Following a stroke there is usually an improvement as the swelling and inflammation around the damaged area of the brain subside. The aim of treatment is to regain as much function as possible so that an individual can be independent and active. This rehabilitation is best achieved using a team, which includes physiotherapists, occupational and speech therapists, as well as doctors. A full recovery is not always possible because dead brain cells cannot be replaced. Therefore greater emphasis is now placed on stroke prevention.

Warning Strokes

Transient ischaemic attacks, commonly called 'warning strokes' or 'little stokes' are, as these names suggest, strokes that last for only a short time but which are significant because they warn that a complete and permanent stroke may occur. The symptoms are similar to a stroke but usually continue for only a few minutes, and never longer than twenty-four hours. Small travelling blood clots from the heart or arteries in the neck temporarily block the blood vessels of the brain causing these transitory symptoms. Taking low dose aspirin prevents these clots from forming and has been shown to reduce the risk of subsequently suffering a stroke.

The danger is that these 'warning strokes' could be ignored because the symptoms are mild and fleeting. As simple and effective treatment is available it is important to report these symptoms to a doctor so that an appropriate assessment can be made and treatment started. Some of the common symptoms are listed below:

- temporary blindness (in one or both eyes);
- double vision;
- difficulty speaking;
- weakness or paralysis of the arm or leg on one side of the body;
- numbness or pins and needles of the arm or leg on one side of the body;
- dizziness;
- impaired mental function;
- recovery is rapid and complete.

Stroke Prevention

During the last three decades there has been a considerable decrease in the number of deaths due to strokes. Although all the reasons for this are not fully understood, an important factor has been a reduction in the risk factors that cause stroke, in particular better detection and treatment of high blood pressure. This is not to suggest complacency, as strokes remain the third most common cause of death after heart disease and cancer. Increasing *age* as well as a *family history* of stroke are risk factors that cannot be altered, but a number of other causes can be rectified. Stroke and heart disease have

many risk factors in common, although their relative importance is different in each case.

High blood pressure is the most important risk factor in causing strokes. Fortunately, even for people in later life, lowering
the blood pressure to normal levels significantly reduces this
risk. Reducing *blood fat* levels, *losing weight*, reducing *alcohol*
intake, and stopping *smoking* should all be considered preventive measures. Strokes are a common problem for *diabetics*,
who should maintain good control of their blood sugar levels.
Of course regular *exercise* is also advisable. *Warning strokes*
must be promptly reported to a doctor so that effective
preventive measures can be implemented. These may range
from taking low dose aspirin, to surgery that clears the narrowed arteries in the neck (carotid endarterectomy).

A Note on Aspirin

There seems to be no doubt that low dose aspirin is beneficial
to people with existing heart disease and for those who have
suffered a 'warning stroke'. It stops the blood from clotting
and blocking narrowed arteries to the heart and brain. The
controversy is whether aspirin offers any benefits to healthy
people. Some studies show that while a small daily dose of
aspirin can reduce the risk of heart attacks, there may be an
increase in strokes due to bleeding in the brain. People with
high blood pressure must be particularly cautious taking
aspirin because of the risk of brain haemorrhage. Aspirin also
has a number of side effects. A common problem is the formation of peptic ulcers and bleeding from the bowel. It is
also possible to be allergic to this drug. Based on the information presently available the widespread use of aspirin by
healthy people is not recommended. If there are a number of
risk factors for heart disease and stroke present, however,
taking aspirin may be beneficial.

Peripheral Vascular Disease/Poor Circulation to the Legs

Narrowing of the arteries in the legs due to atherosclerosis
reduces the supply of blood to those limbs. When the demand
for oxgen carried by the blood is increased during walking

and other exercise, a cramping pain in the calf muscles may be experienced. This pain is rapidly relieved by rest. Other problems resulting from poor circulation include cold feet, thin skin that frequently ulcerates, and in extreme cases gangrene. Medication is of little benefit and most treatment is surgical. This is either performed by inserting a balloon into the artery to stretch and open the narrowed section, or by undergoing a bypass operation to overcome the blockage. Prevention is certainly preferable to either of these procedures.

Prevention

Factors that reduce the formation of fatty plaques in the arteries are again the focus of prevention. Smoking is the major cause of narrowing in the arteries to the legs, and quitting this habit is crucial. Regular exercise is also beneficial because it improves the circulation in the legs. Weight loss relieves the burden of work performed by the legs which are required to carry extra weight. Correcting the other risk factors includes reducing blood fats, maintaining a normal blood pressure and controlling diabetes. These measures have the dual benefits of preventing both heart and peripheral vascular disease.

Heart Failure

Heart failure occurs when the heart lacks the strength to pump a sufficient quantity of blood to satisfy the body's requirements. The fluid that cannot be pumped collects in the lungs and legs, causing breathlessness and swollen ankles. Treatment involves taking fluid tablets that get rid of this excess fluid, and the drug digoxin which helps the heart pump more forcefully.

There are many causes of heart failure, ranging from the over-consumption of alcohol which destroys the muscle of the heart, to the natural wear and tear of the heart valves. However, heart failure is most commonly due to the damage caused by heart attacks and the excessive strain placed on it by uncontrolled high blood pressure. Prevention therefore involves reducing the incidence of heart disease as well as monitoring and treating high blood pressure.

High Blood Pressure

Blood pressure is the pressure in the arteries generated by the heart as it pumps blood around the body. It is represented as two figures, the higher *systolic* measuring the pressure when the heart is contracting and the lower *diastolic* while it is relaxed between beats. Blood pressure varies in response to different activities. It rises with excitement, exercise and stress, returning to normal when these events have passed. Blood pressure is generally higher in older people, but whether this is due to age-related stiffening of the blood vessel walls or to salt in the diet and other lifestyle factors remains controversial. In youth and middle age it is desirable for the blood pressure to be lower than 140/90, while in later life 160/90 is considered normal. Treatment is started if readings are consistently above this level. In the majority of cases the reason for the blood pressure rising is not known, although occasionally kidney disease is to blame.

High blood pressure is often called the 'silent killer' because a person may be unaware that the problem exists. Even when symptoms are noticed they may be vague, with dizziness and headaches being dismissed as normal or due to 'age'. In the absence of any warning the high pressure silently continues to damage the blood vessels and forces the heart to work harder. This can finally lead to a heart attack, heart failure, stroke and kidney disease. Occasionally these tragic complications are the first sign that the blood pressure has been elevated.

It is advisable for older adults to have their blood pressure checked every six months, even if they are feeling well. This is particularly important for people whose parents suffered from high blood pressure or women who had this problem during pregnancy. Measuring blood pressure is a simple, quick and painless procedure that can be performed as part of a general check-up. In this way high blood pressure can be detected and appropriate treatment started before serious complications arise.

In an older person with mildly elevated blood pressure a non-drug treatment alone can be effective. This involves eating foods low in salt, losing excess weight and drinking only small amounts of alcohol. Regular exercise and reducing the level of stress complement these dietary changes. Even if drugs are required an improved lifestyle is still beneficial, as the amount of medication can be reduced to a minimum. This is particularly important for older people who may experience adverse reactions to drugs.

Prevention

Medication controls but does not cure high blood pressure. It is therefore strongly advised that preventive measures are implemented early in life. A number of factors are believed to have a role in preventing high blood pressure, and if corrected, this condition will become less prevalent.

Salt

Eating salty foods can raise blood pressure; a diet low in salt is therefore recommended. Salt should not be added to food, and highly salted processed and snack foods (salami, chips, nuts) should be avoided. Salt reduced products (bread, margarine) are also a better choice than those which contain unnecessary salt.

Increasing the intake of *potassium* is believed to complement the beneficial effects of reducing the intake of salt. Apricots, bananas and tomatoes are foods rich in potassium, but people with poor kidney function must take extra care here, because their bodies may not be able to cope with the extra potassium. Another interesting association between diet and blood pressure is that *vegetarians* are less likely to develop high blood pressure. Their diet contains less saturated fat, and more fruit and vegetables are eaten.

Obesity

People who are overweight are prone to high blood pressure; it is therefore important to maintain a healthy body weight.

Alcohol

In excess of three glasses of alcohol each day causes the blood pressure to rise. As mentioned, however, smaller amounts of alcohol may in fact be beneficial in preventing heart disease.

Exercise

Moderate regular exercise can reduce blood pressure. In addition it helps in weight loss and improves the efficiency of the heart. There are a variety of beneficial exercises, although weight lifting should be avoided as it can cause the blood pressure to rise. Before starting an exercise programme it is advisable that people with high blood pressure undergo a full medical check-up.

Relaxation

Stress and anxiety cause a temporary rise in blood pressure. Although the reverse occurs with relaxation it is debatable whether this actually prevents high blood pressure. Viewing health as an overall state of wellbeing, there is no doubt that a reduction in stress will improve the general health of a tense person who has high blood pressure.

CANCER

Cancer is the second most common cause of death in Australia. The risk of cancer increases with age and it is estimated that 50 per cent of all cancers occur in people over sixty-five. Cancers are not an inevitable part of the ageing process, but a separate group of diseases. It has been estimated that 90 per cent of cancers are related to environmental factors such as smoking and dietary habits. There is therefore plenty of scope for prevention.

Cancer is due to the uncontrolled and disorderly growth of abnormal cells. These cells multiply to reach a reasonable sized 'clump', or *tumour*. Unlike normal cells, they invade other tissues and can spread throughout the body. It is usually many years between the formation of the first abnormal cells and the symptoms of a cancer becoming apparent. The aim of prevention is to stop the initial changes in the cells occurring, for example by not smoking. In addition, even after a cancer has developed the early detection of small tumours before they have spread ensures a successful response to treatment.

In practical terms the scope for completely preventing cancer in later life is limited. Measures to reduce cancer are most effective if introduced at a young age, because there is a significant period of delay, often decades, before the benefits are gained. Smoking, excessive exposure of the skin to sun and an unhealthy diet are factors generally accepted to cause the common cancers. With increased life expectancy some older people may now live long enough to enjoy the advantages of cancer prevention. Another important point here is that older adults can encourage young people to lead healthy lives, by way of example.

Immediate and tangible benefits can be obtained from the early detection of cancer. Too frequently many of the warning signs are accepted as a normal part of ageing, and this allows the cancer to become more advanced. Screening tests such as mammography for breast cancer and Pap smear for cancer of the cervix are useful in detecting disease before the symptoms are evident. Unfortunately, few people in later life have these tests performed, although they are the group at greatest risk. Early detection not only results in a better chance of cure, but the treatment employed is usually less drastic and distressing. Negative results of screening tests can also be beneficial as they are reassuring.

The most common cancers in Australia are those that affect the skin, lungs, bowel, breasts, cervix and the prostate gland. Each will be discussed in detail here.

Skin Cancer

Australia has the highest rate of skin cancer in the world, due mainly to its fair-skinned population living in a sunny climate. This form of cancer becomes increasingly common with advancing age because the skin has been exposed to the damaging rays of the sun for a longer period of time. There are three main types of skin cancer. *Basal cell* and *squamous cell carcinomas* develop on areas of the body most frequently exposed to the sun, particularly the head, neck, forearms and hands. People working outdoors are most at risk. These account for 95 per cent of skin cancers and fortunately are almost always curable if detected early. *Malignant melanomas* spread quickly and are the most lethal form of skin cancer. Although the sun is a factor in causing melanomas, they can arise anywhere on the body and occur in people who work indoors. It is believed that short but intense periods of sun exposure at holidays times increases the risk of indoor workers developing melanomas.

The focus of prevention is to avoid the damaging rays of the sun by sitting in the shade and wearing protective clothing including a wide-brimmed hat. On exposed areas of the skin maximum protection can be achieved by applying a 15+SPF sunscreen. Between 11 am and 3 pm (summer time) the sun's rays are the strongest and most harmful. Therefore it is always advisable to keep out of the sun at this time of the day.

The damaging effects of the sun have become widely known only in the past few years. For this reason many older people, who previously may not have taken the above precautions, may still develop skin cancers. Early detection is relatively easy because the skin is accessible to regular inspection. The three types of skin cancer are described below. If any of these signs are noticed it is advisable to see a doctor.

1. *Basal cell carcinoma* — red, pale or shiny pearl-coloured lump
2. *Squamous cell carcinoma* — red scaly patch, or a sore that does not heal
3. *Melanoma* — spot, freckle or mole that is new; changes shape, size, colour or looks different; or itches or bleeds.

Often dry rough spots called *solar keratosis* are confused with skin cancer, and although they rarely become a cancer, it indicates sun damage has occured. In this case it is wise to carefully search for skin cancers, and to protect the skin from further sun damage.

Lung Cancer

This common cancer is in most cases caused by smoking cigarettes. Quitting reduces the risk by half within five to nine years and after fifteen years is the same as a non-smoker. Therefore even people in later life are able to prevent this fatal disease if they stop smoking. A regular chest x-ray is not recommended; this does not detect the cancer early enough for it to be cured. However a persistent cough, breathlessness or coughing up blood should prompt a smoker to have these symptoms investigated by their doctor. Interestingly, beta-carotene, a derivative of vitamin A, is believed to protect against this form of cancer. It is present in green leafy vegetables (broccoli, spinach), as well as yellow-orange fruit and vegetables (carrots, apricots, cantaloupes).

Bowel Cancer

Bowel cancer is the most common internal malignancy. If detected early it can usually be completely removed surgically. Unfortunately, however, the cancer will often grow to quite an advanced stage before causing symptoms. There are a number of factors that are believed to increase an individual's risk of developing bowel cancer, and by identifying them it can be avoided.

Bowel cancer and food are interrelated. Studies comparing the eating habits and cancer rates in different countries have revealed that the incidence of this cancer is higher in communities where people eat a lot of fat and only a small amount of plant food such as cereals, fruit and vegetables. One way to reduce the risk of cancer is to follow the 'Prudent Diet', which has been formulated by the Anti-Cancer Council:

1. Avoid obesity
2. Cut down on fatty foods.
3. Eat more fibre foods, such as fruits, vegetables and whole grain cereals.
4. Include foods rich in vitamins A and C — they may reduce the risk of cancer.
    Vitamin A — dark green vegetables.
               — yellow fruit and vegetables.
    Vitamin C — citrus fruit, berries, tomato and capsicum.
5. Include cruciferous vegetables which protects against bowel cancer — cabbage, broccoli, brussel sprouts and cauliflower.
6. Be moderate in drinking alcoholic beverages.
7. Be moderate in eating salt-cured, smoked and nitrite-cured foods.

Bowel cancer is due to polyps in the bowel becoming malignant, and finding and removing these growths is an excellent form of prevention. There is a greater chance of bowel cancer and polyps developing in the family members of people who have these tumours, particularly their first degree relatives (mother, father, brother, sister or child). Where there is a history of bowel cancer or polyps in the family, its members should become familiar with ways of detecting this cancer. This includes screening tests and being able to recognize the early signs of disease.

Screening for bowel cancer before the symptoms appear involves a number of procedures. The most simple is for a doctor to examine the rectum (lower end of the bowel) with a gloved finger. Because bowel cancer and polyps frequently bleed the motions can also be tested for the presence of blood (faecal occult blood test). Finally a tube containing a light can be inserted into the bowel, to examine it in greater detail. If the lower section only is checked this is termed sigmoidoscopy, with colonoscopy referring to the more extensive examination of the whole colon. If a polyp is detected while performing these procedures, it can be immediately removed using special instruments, thus preventing bowel cancer.

There is some disagreement as to whether these tests should be performed on everyone in later life or restricted to people who have a high risk of developing bowel cancer. The American Cancer Society recommends a yearly rectal examination and occult blood test for all people over fifty, as well as a sigmoidoscopy examination every few years. The approach in Australia is more conservative, with these procedures being reserved for those at high risk. These checks are usually started at forty years of age. How frequently the tests are performed is best determined by a person's own doctor, who can assess the risks relevant to each individual.

Many people are embarrassed by normal bodily functions, however, it is important to be aware of what is 'normal'. If changes occur these should be reported to a doctor. Blood in the motions is one sign, and should not be dismissed as being due to haemorrhoids. Bleeding always warrants investigation. Likewise, changes in bowel habits should not be ignored, either constipation or diarrhoea, or the sensation of incomplete emptying of the bowel. Stomach pains, weakness and weight loss are common but non-specific complaints that can indicate a bowel problem. Promptly reporting any of these symptoms is likely to result in an early diagnosis and a successful response to treatment.

Breast Cancer

Three years ago I attended a 'Women's Health Day' at the community health centre. It was soon after my sister had her breast cancer operation and I was concerned that I may have the same problem. A lady doctor first took a smear test, which surprised me as I thought only young women needed this examination. Next a film was shown on how to examine the breasts for cancer. A doctor checked my breasts but did not find any lumps. Because my sister had cancer it was recommended that I go back to my own G.P. to have a mammography test. The first X-ray was normal but the next one, two months ago, showed a suspicious lump that did prove to be cancer. The surgeon removed it and because the lump was small he feels that there is now nothing to worry about. Another surprise for me was that only the lump was removed and my breast remains the same as before the operation.

Emma (62)

Breast cancer affects one in fifteen Australian women at some stage in their life. The disease itself is feared, and the prospects of treatment are often threatening. Recently there has been a significant change in attitude towards breast cancer, with a greater emphasis on prevention and less radical surgery being performed whenever possible. If breast cancer is detected early the prospects of a cure are good, and the treatment is usually simpler and less drastic. The risk factors for breast cancer are:

• age — more common in older women;
• family history — mother, sister, aunt with breast cancer;
• early menstruation, late menopause;
• motherhood — no children, first child born when aged thirty plus;
• obesity and high fat diet.

There are no known causes of breast cancer, however a women's risk of developing it is increased if her mother, sister

or aunt had breast cancer. There is also an association between breast cancer and obesity, particularly if the diet is high
in fat; yet another reason to choose low fat foods. As a woman
can do relatively little to prevent breast cancer from developing, there has been much campaigning for its early detection.
In Sweden and England there is widespread support to screen
all women for breast cancer. Australia has a number of pilot
studies underway and breast cancer screening is likely to start
soon. Until this occurs, women at risk should consider being
checked regularly. This can be done by their own doctor or
at special clinics.

The three methods of screening for breast cancer are breast
self-examination, physical examination of the breast, and
mammography. These tests complement each other and all
three should be employed together. They aim to detect small
cancers, at the stage before they have spread.

Breast Self-examination

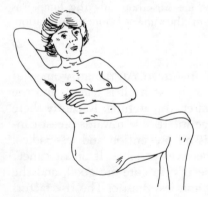
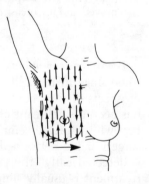

Position for breast self
examination (BSE)

The area to be covered
by examination

FIGURE 7.2   Breast self-examination.

A regular systematic examination of the breast allows a
woman to become familiar with her own breasts and notice
any changes. The recommended method of examination is
described in Figure 7.2. Ideally it should be performed once
a month, preferably after a period, or in post-menopausal
women on a convenient day (the first day of each month is

easy to remember). The aim is to detect small thickenings or lumps in the breast. Other signs to look for are a change in shape of the breast, and tenderness, discharge or 'turning in' of the nipple. Although the majority do not turn out to be cancerous, all breast lumps should be examined by a doctor.

Physical Examination of the Breast

A yearly examination of a woman's breasts by her doctor, or other specially trained personnel, has been shown to be beneficial in detecting early breast cancer. Often this examination can be done in conjunction with a routine smear test.

Mammography

Mammography is a special X-ray of the breast used to detect cancer. As a screening test it has the advantage of being able to identify lumps that cannot be felt. Half of all breast cancers occur in women older than fifty, and mammography has been demonstrated to be effective in reducing the number who die from breast cancer. It is recommended that routine mammography be performed every one to two years in all women aged fifty and older. It is debatable whether those in the forty to forty-nine age group benefit from routine mammography, and it is generally not recommended for women under forty.

The risk from radiation used to X-ray the breast is small, and has been calculated to be equivalent to the risk involved in travelling 200 miles by air or thirty miles in a car. It is important to emphasize that no single method is infallible and that if a lump is felt, even if mammography is normal, further tests may be required. These may involve removing the whole lump surgically or using a fine needle to take a small sample of tissue which is then examined for cancer. This latter method is simpler and does not require admission to hospital.

The medical advantages of screening for breast cancer in older women are well recognized. At the present time it appears to be the only way to control and reduce this common cancer. In the near future mammography is likely to be more widely available in Australia, but its success will depend on the amount of money governments allocate to the scheme, and how women themselves accept this form of testing.

Cancer of the Cervix

The cervix is situated at the lower end of the womb and, being easily accessible by vaginal examination, cancer of the a cervix can be detected early by a Pap smear test. This is a simple and painless procedure involving the gentle removal of cells from the cervix which are then examined under a microscope. As it takes many years for the cancer to evolve, early pre-cancerous changes in the cells can be identified and after appropriate treatment a woman is completely cured. If routine smear tests are not done the cancer remains un-detected and serious complications arise.

Although this is an almost perfect screening test, women continue to die from cancer of the cervix. This is mainly because some older women do not know that smear tests are still necessary in later life, or because these are not done regularly. A common problem is that these women gave birth to their children decades ago, before a routine smear test be-came accepted medical practice, they may therefore simply not know about smear tests. Embarrassment is another prob-lem that can be overcome by discussing these fears and misgivings with a doctor. As is pointed out by the Anti-Cancer Council, 'nobody has ever died from embarrassment, but women who didn't know about smear tests have died of cancer of the cervix'.

It is recommended that all women have smear tests every two years. Post-menopausal women, as well as those who may no longer be sexually active, should be tested. It is con-venient, and recommended, that a woman having a smear test should also have a vaginal examination. This will reveal if there is enlargement of the ovaries and uterus. Vaginal bleeding, particularly after menopause or following inter-course, is not normal and a woman should report this to her doctor.

Apart from early detection there is no known way to prevent cancer of the cervix, although, because a virus infection is suspected, sexual activity in younger years probably has some influence. As with lung cancer, beta-carotene may offer some degree of protection from this cancer.

Prostate Cancer

There are no known causes for cancer of the prostate, however it seems to be associated with a high fat diet. Growth of the cancer is stimulated by the male hormone testosterone and as cholesterol is used to produce it, some doctors believe that the excess amount of fat in the diet increases the production of this hormone. Prostate cancer is particularly common in older men, who in every other way are healthy 'survivors'.

The symptoms of an enlarged prostate are the same whether it is due to cancer or a benign growth of the gland. Difficulty or pain when passing urine, and frequency of urination (during the day or night) are common problems. The only way to detect early prostate cancer is for a doctor to perform a yearly rectal examination.

OBESITY

After retirement I began to feel tired and my vision seemed to be getting worse. In the beginning I thought it would pass once I adjusted to not working, and was surprised when the doctor told me I had diabetes. He said if I lost weight by exercising and eating healthy foods, I would probably not need tablets or insulin. For years I had been promising myself to lose weight but this was the 'push' I needed. In fact it was not as hard as I had thought. There was no longer the problem of business lunches and we shopped at the market for our fruit and vegetables. It became an enjoyable outing. Being retired there is also more time to exercise. Although the loss of weight is slow I am confident my goal weight can be achieved.

Arthur (62)

It is incorrect to assume that because many people gain weight as they become older, this is a normal part of ageing. Being overweight is the result of eating more than the body requires, with the excess being stored as fat. Older adults tend to gain weight because they are often less active, and the body's metabolism naturally slows with age. The solution therefore is to eat less and exercise more.

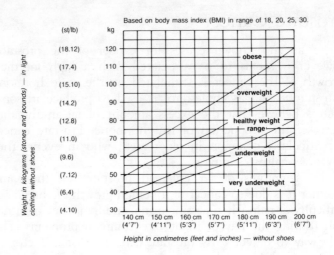

FIGURE 7.3 Ideal weight ranges.

The ideal weight ranges for different heights are listed in Figure 7.3. People who are more than 20 per cent overweight are classified as being obese. Pinching the fat below the waist between the thumb and index finger is another simple check. If it is wider than 2.5 cm (1 inch), the person is overweight.

The extra body fat is a risk to health. The medical problems associated with obesity include:

- heart disease;
- stroke;
- high blood pressure;
- high blood fat levels;
- diabetes (non-insulin dependent);
- cancer (breast, colon and prostate);
- arthritis and back problems;
- gall bladder disease;
- surgical complications.

Weight loss can be successfully achieved by reducing the amount of food eaten, as well as becoming more active. To ensure that healthy habits remain permanent there must also be a change in lifestyle and behaviour. These important aspects of weight loss are explained below.

Healthy Eating

To lose weight it is essential to eat a balanced and nutritious diet containing a wide variety of foods. It also involves limiting foods that contain fat and sugar; these are high in calories (kilojoules) but have little nutritional value. Aim for a slow but steady weight loss of $\frac{1}{2}$–1 kg each week, which over a number of months adds up to a significant reduction in body fat. This also ensures that the new healthy habits become established and the weight loss is permanent. Practical information on a sensible eating plan for people in later life is explained in Chapter 4.

There are a number of problems with crash and fad diets which offer superficially simple solutions to overweight people. Weight loss on such diets is usually temporary; the weight is regained as soon as 'normal' eating practices are resumed. These diets can also be too strict, and may lack important nutrients. When the body is subjected to a severe 'starvation' diet, its metabolism slows down in an attempt to conserve energy. Losing weight therefore becomes even more difficult. Tablets and operations to lose weight are also unacceptable due to their sometimes serious side effects. It is preferable to accept healthy eating as a normal part of daily life rather than a dieting ordeal. Eating should remain a pleasure, and at the same time a desirable weight should be maintained.

Increase Activity

Exercise 'burns up' some of the energy obtained from food. It has the added benefit of counteracting the normal slowing of the metabolism by increasing the body's metabolic rate for up to twenty-four hours after exercise. More food can be eaten so that there is unlikely to be a lack of nutrients, a problem that can occur if the diet is too strict.

A wide variety of exercises are available. Brisk walking is simple, effective and within the abilities of almost everyone. In addition to periods of exercise, increasing everyday activity, such as walking to the shops rather than driving, improve fitness and prevent weight being gained. Turn back to Chapter 3 for a fuller discussion of the benefits of exercise.

Changing Behaviour

Many people know in theory what to do to lose weight but fail to put it into practice. Changing behaviour is a common-sense approach that enables healthy eating and exercise to be successfully implemented. Dietary habits are learnt, therefore an overweight person is more likely to lose and then maintain his or her desirable weight if new and healthier habits are learnt. Below are listed a number of hints that can help to achieve a normal weight.

- Eat less and exercise more;
- Moderate changes in eating and exercise will allow them to be permanently integrated into the daily routine;
- Change attitudes towards food and dieting — consider eating healthily forever rather than strict dieting for a short period of time;
- Think positively about all the benefits of healthy eating rather than dwell on being deprived of unhealthy foods;
- Set realistic goals and indulge in a reward (other than food) when these are achieved;
- Lose weight slowly — $\frac{1}{2}$–1 kg per week;
- Check body weight each week to monitor loss and prevent the weight being regained when the goal weight has been achieved;
- Become familiar with the energy (kilojoule) value of foods;
- Keep a diary that records the food eaten, its energy (kilojoule) value, and feelings at the time of eating, for example hungry, bored;
- Start eating only when hungry and arrange activities other than eating to alleviate feelings of boredom, frustration and tension;
- Eat three meals and avoid unhealthy snacks between meals;
- Eat the meals in one place; sit and take time to enjoy the food;
- Don't do other activities while eating, such as watching television;
- Eat slowly, put down the knife and fork while chewing;
- Shop after a meal and use a shopping list to stop impulse buying;

- Avoid having unhealthy foods in the house (even for visitors);
- Setbacks are common and if there is a relapse learn from the experience rather than feeling guilty, disheartened or bingeing;
- Encouragement from family and friends is beneficial;
- Exercise and mealtime should both be enjoyable.

DIABETES

Diabetes can be best understood by following the sequence of events that occur when a person eats a meal. The sugars and starches in food are first converted to glucose which the body can utilize. In response to the food, insulin is released from the pancreas and moves glucose from the bloodstream into cells where it can be used for energy. Diabetes is a disorder in which either insufficient insulin is produced or it is ineffective, causing the level of glucose in the blood to rise. Diabetes is identified by these high blood glucose levels.

There are two types of diabetes. *Insulin dependent diabetes* can occur at any age but usually young people are affected. They lack insulin and therefore are required to inject it for the remainder of their lives. The more common type is *non-insulin dependent diabetes*, and this usually develops later in life. Five per cent of people over sixty have this form of diabetes. Although insulin is produced it is ineffective in lowering blood glucose. Treatment involves weight reduction, exercise and a sensible diet, but if these measures are insufficient then medication may also be prescribed.

A less well known disorder of glucose metabolism is *impaired glucose tolerance*, which also occurs in older adults. There are usually no symptoms and therefore the diagnosis can only be made by measuring blood glucose levels. This condition borders on non-insulin dependent diabetes because the amount of glucose in the blood is elevated. Not surprisingly, these people are likely to become diabetic in the future. They are also more likely to suffer from heart disease and strokes. Treatment involves lifestyle changes such as losing weight, exercise and healthy eating.

The classical symptoms of diabetes are weight loss, thirst and passing urine frequently, while non-specific feelings of tiredness, blurred vision and infections can also occur. Returning blood glucose to normal levels will alleviate these unpleasant symptoms. After many years diabetics may develop complications. Atherosclerosis is accelerated causing heart disease, stroke and reduced circulation to the legs. Poor vision, kidney and nerve damage are other long-term problems. These complications are less likely if the diabetes is well controlled.

Prevention

The degree to which insulin and non-insulin dependent diabetes can be prevented is vastly different, despite the fact that heredity is a major factor in both cases. There are no known means of preventing insulin dependent diabetes (which is thought to be caused by a disorder of the immune system triggered by a virus or other agents), however, lifestyle factors such as obesity, a poor diet and sedentary living can give rise to non-insulin dependent diabetes in genetically susceptible adults. This form of diabetes is therefore amenable to prevention by an improvement in lifestyle. Maintaining a *healthy body weight* and avoiding obesity are the most important factors in prevention. Part and parcel of this is eating a *sensible diet*. There is some evidence to suggest that a high fibre diet may be beneficial, although this remains contentious. *Stress* is also thought to have a role in causing diabetes but this too has yet to be proven. *Exercise* is the final factor which is believed to have a protective effect.

Diabetes Australia estimates that there are now as many as 500 000 people suffering from diabetes, of whom 250 000 are undiagnosed and are therefore unaware of their condition. Because of the hereditary nature of diabetes it is particularly important for people with a family history of diabetes to be checked. Routine testing of urine (or blood) will detect diabetes and treatment will not only improve a person's present health but also prevent long-term complications.

Preventing long-term complications is also a strong incentive to maintain good control of the diabetes. As well as the self-monitoring of sugar levels, regular check-ups in which a doctor screens for these problems is advisable. Of particular importance is an annual eye examination as early detection of eye problems allows them to be promptly treated. Foot disorders can be another potential source of concern and diabetics should attend a podiatrist for all aspects of foot care.

MENOPAUSE

After my fiftieth birthday I felt down and irritable. At night I would suddenly feel hot and throw off the blankets. My husband seemed confused and was not understanding. I did not know whether it was 'change of life' or being depressed approaching a new decade in my life. I discussed it with my mother who said she never even noticed her own menopause. At the next routine visit to the gynaecologist for a smear test I mentioned these problems to her. She assured me they would improve with hormone treatment. Almost immediately the flushes disappeared and I slept soundly. My husband also commented that now I was much happier.

Peta (51)

Menopause is a normal event in the reproductive lifecycle of women and is marked by the cessation of menstruation. Most Australian women have their menopause between the ages of forty-five and fifty-five, with the years after menopause now representing one third of their lifetime. Fortunately, much of the apprehension and ignorance associated with menopause has disappeared and older women no longer have to endure unpleasant menopausal symptoms, as effective relief is readily available.

The actual period of transition spans two to five years. During this time ovarian function diminishes, with less of the female hormones oestrogen and progesterone being produced. This results in the loss of fertility and changes to other tissues that are affected by these hormones. A popular misconception is that most women will suffer distressing menopausal symptoms that require treatment. In fact the majority either do not notice any change, or their symptoms are minor. Only 15 per cent of women describe menopause as severely distressing. The main concerns of menopausal women are hot flushes, vaginal and urinary problems, emotional changes and osteoporosis.

Hot flushes are the hallmark of an uncomfortable menopause. These women experience a sudden hot sensation, accompanied by a blotchy, red flushing of the skin and sweats. Frequently hot flushes and sweats occur at night, disturbing sleep. The lack of oestrogen also causes the skin of the vagina to become thin and dry. This can result in vaginal irritation and discomfort, particularly during intercourse. A lubricant, such as K-Y gel, or an oestrogen cream will usually alleviate this problem. The hormonal changes of menopause usually do not alter a woman's sex drive. If, however, intercourse becomes painful due to the lack of vaginal lubrication, sex may be avoided for this reason. Similar changes occur to the urinary system which is adjacent to the vagina, causing the frequent passing of urine and bladder infections. In addition, the reduced amounts of hormones can weaken the pelvic muscles, which support the bladder and womb, allowing them to prolapse. This can result in urinary incontinence.

Other menopausal symptoms include headaches, dizziness, tiredness, palpitations, nausea and bloatedness. The female hormone oestrogen is also essential in maintaining healthy bones and after menopause osteoporosis often occurs. These weaker bones can break more easily and many doctors advocate replacement of oestrogen to prevent this irreversible loss of bone.

The emotional feelings at the time of menopause are varied. Some women experience no problems while others are depressed, irritable and lose confidence. A woman's changing role and the loss of her ability to bear children may require a significant emotional adjustment. It is often at this time that children become independent and leave the family home. A mother may no longer feel useful or appreciated by her family, the so called 'empty nest syndrome'. It is difficult to separate whether the hormonal, physical or psychological changes occurring are contributing to these feelings, but more than likely all have some influence. It is important, therefore, to consider all the possible alternatives for resolving such feelings, and not to rely solely on hormone replacement.

A woman who leads a healthy, active and fulfilling life is likely to overcome the challenges that confront her during menopause. Regular exercise, not smoking and sensible eating, particularly an adequate intake of calcium to strengthen bones, remain important for good health and well-being. Time set aside for rest and relaxation will enhance the quality of life.

Regular check-ups are advisable. In addition to a thorough examination, screening for breast cancer and smear tests should be performed routinely. Many women will also benefit from practising pelvic exercises, which strengthen the pelvic muscles preventing incontinence and a prolapse (see Appendix 1).

Emotional problems can be tackled by obtaining support from family and friends. By expressing her feelings a woman informs other people that she is experiencing difficulties. Knowing this they can comfort and assist her. Professional help is also available, either from a doctor or special menopause clinics.

Hormone Replacement Therapy

The pendulum of opinion regarding hormone replacement after menopause has swung between two extremes. Previously, in more chauvinistic times, many male doctors considered menopausal women neurotic and their symptoms as not requiring relief. At the other extreme, some now treat menopause as a 'hormone deficiency disease', the implication being that all women should have their hormones artificially replaced. A more sensible approach is to use hormone replacement therapy when the benefits obtained from such treatment exceed the disadvantages. Replacing the hormones eases menopausal symptoms but is not an anti-ageing cure.

The advantage of hormone replacement therapy is that it reverses most of the changes associated with menopause. Within a short period of time, a woman's hot flushes and night sweats will disappear. Vaginal and urinary symptoms are relieved by either the local application of an oestrogen cream or by taking tablets containing this hormone. Emotional and mood changes can also improve with hormone replacement.

Osteoporosis and heart disease are common diseases in later life which can also be prevented by hormone replacement. Taking oestrogen tablets for five to ten years after menopause will stop the leaching of calcium from bone that results in osteoporosis. Despite hormones being the most effective method of preventing this disorder, bone that has already been lost will not be replaced. Before menopause women have less heart disease than men due to the natural protective effects of the female hormones. This benefit is lost after menopause. At present the balance of evidence suggests that hormone replacement therapy restores this advantage and reduces heart disease in older women.

A number of the side effects of hormone replacement therapy are similar to those experienced by women taking the oral contraceptive pill. Nausea and breast soreness can occur, but the continuation of menstruation is the most common reason for refusing this treatment. Medical problems such as a rise in blood pressure and increased blood clotting make it necessary for women contemplating hormone replacement to be assessed by their doctor. There has been a considerable amount of research to establish if continuing to take hormones after menopause adds to the risk of developing cancer. While there is no increase in breast cancer, it has been found that oestrogen causes cancer of the womb. Fortunately this risk is removed by the addition of another female hormone (progesterone) for ten to fourteen days each month. Oestrogen stimulates the lining of the womb to grow, while the progesterone produces shedding of this growth thereby expelling any cancer cells that may have developed. Although continued menstruation may be inconvenient, it is essential in preventing cancer of the womb.

As mentioned, before starting treatment women should undergo a full medical examination including blood pressure check, breast and pelvic examination as well as a smear test. Those with medical problems such as high blood pressure, heart disease, cancer or diabetes have to be particularly cautious and discuss the effects of hormone replacement therapy with their doctor. Tablets are the most common way of replacing the hormones, although occasionally creams alone are enough to relieve vaginal discomfort. An alternative is the implantation of small pellets under the skin that slowly release their hormones over a period of months. The most recent innovation is a patch containing oestrogen that is absorbed through the skin.

The Male Menopause

This topic has not received the same amount of attention as

the female menopause and consequently much less is known about it. Even the existence of a male menopause is disputed, which is understandable as the term 'menopause' cannot truly be applied to men as they do not menstruate! If 'change of life' is used then there is some evidence to suggest that a few men may experience similar symptoms to women. Hot flushes, depression and anxiety have been reported but usually occur ten years after the female menopause. Whether these are due to a reduction in the amount of male hormones or a reaction to an older man's changing role is difficult to determine. There does not appear to be an abrupt or significant decrease in the level of the male hormone testosterone and therefore hormone replacement therapy is not an accepted form of treatment. Career, health and relationships frequently alter in later life and may be the explanations for these changes. Further research needs to be done to find out more about the 'male menopause'.

ARTHRITIS

Recently my right knee became painful. I was very annoyed when the doctor, in an off-hand and arrogant manner, told me that old people had to expect these inconveniences. I replied that this could not possibly be true as the other knee was the same age but not painful. My new doctor referred me to a physiotherapist and the pain has almost gone.

Alex (72)

Arthritis occurs when joints become inflamed, causing pain, swelling and stiffness. It is the most common chronic condition in later life, with half the people at retirement age being affected. Although there are over a hundred different types of arthritis, those most prevalent in older adults are osteoarthritis, rheumatoid arthritis and gout.

Many people over sixty years of age have *osteoarthritis*, but fortunately it does not always cause discomfort. Although the exact cause of osteoarthritis is unknown, it is thought to be due to joints accumulating a lifetime of 'wear and tear'. Other factors that contribute to joints becoming arthritic include subjecting them to repeated trauma and excessive mechanical stress. Being overweight, sustaining an injury and overuse are examples of the extra demands they may have to endure. Heredity factors are also significant in predisposing an individual to arthritis.

Normally the cartilage that covers the bone ends is smooth and rubbery. Osteoarthritis is the result of degeneration and loss of this protective cartilage which becomes worn, frayed and irregular. Pain, stiffness and in extreme cases difficulty moving the joints may be experienced as the degenerative process progresses. Those subjected to the greatest mechanical stress are most affected. These include the weight-bearing joints such as the hips, knees, feet and spine. Involvement of the hands is usually at the base of the thumb and the last finger joints, which can interfere with everyday activities.

Rheumatoid arthritis differs from osteoarthritis in a number of ways. Usually the smaller joints of the hands and feet become inflamed, and although it can occur in later life rheumatoid arthritis is more likely to start in youth or middle age. It is also a generalized disease, affecting a number of organs such as the lungs and blood vessels as well as the joints. The cause is not known but it is believed to be due to the person's own immune system attacking these tissues.

Gout is due to excessive amounts of uric acid in the body and the painful attacks of arthritis are the result of sharp uric acid crystals forming in the joints. The big toe is the classical site for gout but other joints can be involved.

Prevention

Arthritis has for centuries attracted a variety of folk remedies, ranging from special diets which eliminate 'acid foods' to the common practice of wearing a copper bracelet. Claims that these treatments prevent or cure arthritis have not been scientifically substantiated. There is no known means of preventing rheumatoid arthritis and the emphasis is therefore on minimizing joint damage. Fortunately some measures can be adopted to avoid or slow the development of osteoarthritis.

There are a number of ways people can keep their joints functioning and healthy. Regular use and exercise nourishes and lubricates joints, ensuring that their full range of movements are maintained. It also strengthens the muscles around a joint, giving them greater stability and protection against injury. Following an accident or injury early treatment and allowing an adequate time for complete healing are essential if subsequent arthritis is to be avoided. Another strategy for those who want to care for their joints is to protect them from mechanical stress and trauma. Jarring activities and over-use places excessive strain on joints causing damage which can eventually lead to osteoarthritis. Often these activities will cause pain, a warning signal that the joint is over-stressed and that the activity should be stopped. Rhythmic moderate exercises such as walking and swimming generally do not cause problems. Weight loss is also recommended for a person who is overweight. The extra weight is a burden for the joints of the legs and back.

Back care warrants special consideration. Maintaining a good posture while sitting, standing and sleeping is vital if back problems are to be avoided. Correct lifting techniques, which involve bending the knees while the back remains straight, are simple but effective preventive measures. Exercises such as swimming strengthen the back muscles, which support and protect the spine for injury.

Osteoarthritis will never be totally preventable until its precise cause is found. The next practical step is to ensure that people with arthritis do not lose their independence or become disabled. Most medical treatment is directed towards achieving this objective and involves relieving the pain and restoring function to arthritic joints. Simple pain killers such as paracetamol and aspirin are often sufficient to ease osteoarthritic pain. If the joint is severely inflamed then stronger anti-inflammatory arthritis tablets can be taken. In addition to medication there are a number of physical remedies such as physiotherapy and hydrotherapy (exercises in a warm pool) that can provide relief. Practical advice and special equipment, to make everyday living easier, can be obtained from an occupational therapist. Frequently these physical treatments are neglected and tablets are the only form of treatment offered. The final option to restore function in a severely damaged joint is to operate and replace it with a new artificial joint. This form of surgery is commonly performed on the hip and knee. Al-though a drastic form of treatment these operations enable independence to be regained.

Gout, like heart disease, obesity and high blood pressure is associated with an affluent lifestyle. A person who wishes to prevent gout should avoid the risk factors associated with these ailments. In addition, it is important to maintain a healthy body weight and choose a sensible diet. Foods rich in purines, a precursor of uric acid, should not be eaten. These include organ meats (liver, brains sweetmeats, kidneys) and certain tinned fish (sardines, anchoves, herring). Sudden changes in eating habits and crash diets can also bring on an attack of gout. Only moderate amounts of alcohol are advisable. If the level of uric acid remains unacceptably high then allopurinol tablets, which will reduce it to normal, may be recommended.

The Arthritis Foundation can provide further information, advice and support to people with arthritis.

OSTEOPOROSIS

I had never heard of osteoporosis until I fell and broke my wrist. The doctor explained a number of different treatments but I have never liked taking tablets. I chose to drink more milk and to cut down on salty foods. Deciding which exercise was difficult as I have arthritis in my knees. The 'Fabulous Fifties' water aerobics at the local pool is not only good for my bones and general fitness, but lots of fun.

Hilda (66)

Osteoporosis was until recently a term heard only in medical circles. It has now joined cholestrol, atherosclerosis and fibre as a word used in all sections of the community. This reflects the increasing incidence of the problem in older people. It is a common disorder, affecting one third of women after menopause and to a lesser extent older men. Natural ageing causes a gradual loss of bone in both men and women. This loss is rapid in the first five years after a woman's menopause, as decreasing levels of the female hormones allows calcium to leave the bones. This is why the problem is most common in older women.

The literal meaning of osteoporosis is 'porous bones', and it is caused by calcium loss. This thinning weakens the bones which are then more easily fractured. The wrist, spine and hip are most commonly broken. A fractured hip can result in serious complications for an older person, emphasizing the importance of preventing osteoporosis.

Prevention begins with identifying those people who have an increased chance of developing osteoporosis. The risk factors include:

— female sex
— family history of osteoporosis
— small thin frame
— European or Asian
— early menopause (before forty-five years)
— drugs e.g. cortisone, some aluminium antacids
— low calcium diet*
— sedentary lifestyle*
— alcohol*
— cigarette smoking*
— caffeine (more than three of coffee a day)*
— lack of vitamin D (from sunlight, oils, yellow vegetables)*
— food: high protein, high salt, high fibre*

Sometimes it is only after suffering a fracture that a woman becomes aware that she has osteoporosis. X-rays are not good indicators of the problem; they reveal thinning of the bones only when one third has already been lost. Clearly this is unsatisfactory for early detection and prevention. Densitometry, a new safe technique that accurately measures bone density is now available. At present there are only a few machines in Australia, but this is likely to change with the recognition of osteoporosis as a significant health problem. Ideally all women at risk should be screened at menopause.

Osteoporosis is difficult to treat once it is established and so prevention is essential. A number of the lifestyle risk factors can be altered (those marked with an asterisk), and form the basis for preventing the condition. The earlier these measures are implemented the stronger a women's bones will be when she starts menopause.

Regular Weight Bearing Exercise

During exercise the bones are being 'used', which strengthens them and prevents the loss of calcium. Walking, dancing and tennis are some examples but all forms of activity are beneficial. Ideally exercise should be performed for thirty minutes three times each week, with adequate warm-up and cool-down periods (see Chapter 3).

Hormone Replacement Therapy (HRT)

Replacing the female hormone oestrogen after menopause is the most effective way of halting the rapid loss of bone that occurs in older women. Combining calcium supplements with hormone replacement has also been shown to be effective. These measures are particularly important for women who have an early menopause (younger than forty-five years) whether naturally or after surgery that removes the ovaries. Other benefits and risks of hormone replacement are discussed in the previous section which deals with menopause (pp 207–8). As mentioned, hormones are unable to restore bone already lost.

Calcium

Calcium is essential for healthy bones. The recommended daily requirement of calcium for older women is 1000 mg which is 200 mg more than premenopausal women. Surveys have revealed that the average daily intake of calcium is only 500–700 mg which is significantly less than the recommended amount. One reason for this is that many people exclude dairy foods from their diet in order to lose weight and lower blood cholesterol levels. This practice is incorrect and unhealthy. It is preferable to consume reduced fat milk, yoghurt and cheese as these are high in calcium but low in calories and fat.

The main dietary sources of calcium are milk and milk products. The daily requirement of calcium can be obtained from eating two serves of dairy foods plus a healthy balanced diet. Other food sources are listed on pages 104–5, where the daily requirements are also given.

Calcium supplements may be indicated if the dietary intake of calcium is low. It is preferable to take them on an empty stomach before bedtime.

Lifestyle Changes

A diet high in salt, alcohol and caffeine has been shown to be associated with an excessive loss of calcium in the urine.

This results in less calcium being available to the bones and promotes osteoporosis. These lifestyle changes help to prevent a number of other common diseases such as heart disease, high blood pressure and certain cancers.

FALLS AND FRACTURES

Falls in later life cause unnecessary injury and suffering. Older people have a tendency to overbalance and fall due to a natural decline in the function of their nervous system. A less accurate sense of the body's position, slower reflexes and poor co-ordination contribute to this unsteadiness. Combined with weaker muscles and unstable arthritic joints, older adults are more vulnerable to trip and stumble. There is a greater reliance on vision to maintain balance and if this also fails then the falls can become frequent.

Fortunately most falls are not serious and no injury is sustained. When a person is hurt, apart from cuts and bruises, fractures are the most worrying complication, and these are likely to occur if the bones are thin and osteoporotic.

A single accidental fall or trip is not an ominous event. It is often caused by an environmental hazard such as a slippery floor or dim lighting. Half the number of falls that occur are in this category. Further falls can be prevented by identifying and rectifying the environmental hazard that contributed to the accident. Modifying a home and incorporating into its design features that promote safety is essential. A number of suggestions are listed in Table 7.1. The fear of falling can be overcome by remaining active. This not only maintains confidence but also increases fitness, strengthens muscles and improves joint flexibility. It is not a good idea to adopt a 'safe' and sedentary way of life; inactivity will only erode confidence.

Repeated falls are often due to ill health and indicate the need for a thorough medical assessment. Heart disease, neurological disorders and side effects from drugs are the most common causes. A number of these can be corrected and so further falls prevented. Following a stroke or a prolonged period of bed rest due to ill health, rehabilitation is frequently required to strengthen muscles and improve walking. Drug side effects should be closely monitored by the prescribing

TABLE 7.1 Preventing falls in later life

The environment

- Stairs — handrails, well lit, clearly marked step edge, short flights of stairs.
- Furniture — chairs: correct height for easier standing;
    — bed: correct height so that feet touch the ground when sitting on the side of the bed;
    — furniture arranged so as not to be obstructive.
- Storage space — avoid using places that require stretching or climbing to reach them.
- Floors — avoid slippery and uneven surfaces;
    — remove throw rugs and loose objects on the floor.
- Cords and wires — reposition to prevent tripping.
- Lighting — light next to bed and over stairs;
    — night light if required (e.g. going to the toilet).
- Bathroom — non-slip mat;
    — rails and seat if necessary.
- Footwear — comfortable and well-fitting (beware of loose and worn slippers).
- Temperature — warm house to 18°C; low body temperature (hypothermia) is associated with falls.
- Aids-walking stick.
- Public transport — safe design.
- Alarm system for summoning help.

The person

- Neurological disorders — stroke/TIA (warning stroke), epilepsy, Parkinson's disease, dementia.
- Heart disease — low blood pressure, irregular heart beat, heart valve abnormalities.
- Drugs — sedatives, antidepressants;
    — alcohol;
    — tablets for treating blood pressure and diabetes.
- Disorders of the muscles and joints
    — arthritis (e.g. unstable knee joint);
    — weakness of muscles due to inactivity (prolonged bed rest).
- Poor vision.

doctor. A number of commonly used medications can cause dizziness when a person stands abruptly. If the medication cannot be stopped or the dose reduced it is advisable to move slowly when changing position. For example, after lying it is preferable to sit on the side of the bed for a few moments before standing.

Poor vision is another disability which causes falls and can often be easily corrected by appropriate specialist treatment. Finally, if there is the possibility of not being able to summon help after a fall, friends and neighbours could call regularly, or a person can carry a small telephone-linked alarm system which is activated in an emergency.

FOOT CARE

It is estimated that in a lifetime people walk 120 000 kilometres; it is therefore not surprising that after many years of faithful service feet can become painful. Many complaints are simply due to the normal wear and tear of physical activity. With proper foot care a number of problems can be prevented.

Extra weight is an unnecessary burden for the feet to carry and this added strain can be avoided by maintaining a healthy weight. Feet should also be kept clean by regular washing in warm soapy water. Careful drying between the toes is especially important as dampness contributes to tinea. A small amount of methylated spirits (applied using a cotton bud) or foot powder will ensure that this area is dry. After the feet have been washed and dried, a cream can be applied to soften scaly or cracked skin (commonly on the heel).

Correct cutting of the toe nails is essential. The nail should be cut straight across, level with the end of the toe, and the sharp edges gently filed. The side of the nail must never be cut away, as this can result in an ingrown toenail.

Buying a pair of comfortable and well-fitting shoes is a worthwhile investment. Check there is adequate room for the toes and that the shoes are flexible at the ball of the foot but have a firm arch support. It is best not to wear slippers for long periods of time as they tend to encourage shuffling and do not provide adequate support. The recent popularity of running shoes means that comfort is no longer excluded by the trends in fashion. Low heels and a non-slip sole also add stability to walking. Socks are also important. Cotton or woollen socks are preferable as they absorb perspiration and stretch with foot movements.

The feet are the furthermost outpost of the body and therefore the most vulnerable to circulatory problems. People must quit smoking as it seriously interferes with circulation. Socks with tight elastic tops and sitting cross-legged can also block the flow of blood. Regular exercise is beneficial as it improves circulation to the feet.

Diabetics are prone to foot problems, especially poor circulation and impaired sensation in the feet. Even minor injuries should receive immediate attention as they can escalate and become serious. It is important for diabetics to regularly attend a podiatrist, even if it is only to have their feet checked and nails cut.

Podiatrists are qualified to treat many foot disorders such as corns, callouses and bunions. Self-treatment with a knife, caustic chemicals or pads is not advisable. Too often comfortable healthy feet are taken for granted, even though they can have a dramatic impact on a person's ability to remain active, mobile and independent.

LUNG DISEASE

The discovery of antibiotics has dramatically improved the treatment of many lung infections. Tuberculosis is now a relatively rare disease and the chest X-ray screening programme of the 1950s has been relegated to medical history. Diseases related to smoking, however, have become more prevalent and are a major community health problem.

The association between *lung cancer* and smoking is well established. *Chronic bronchitis* and *emphysema* are similarly caused by smoking, and because the amount of damage is proportional to the number of cigarettes smoked, heavy smokers are more severely affected. Cigarette smoke contains a number of noxious substances including nicotine, tar and irritating particles. These damage the breathing passages (bronchial tubes) and thin walled air sacs deep in the lungs. The inflammation of the bronchial tubes results in coughing and wheezing, the symptoms of chronic bronchitis. Emphysema is caused by the breakdown of the tiny air sacs. It is a serious condition as the destruction of lung tissue reduces the amount of oxygen able to enter the bloodstream.

Smokers are also more likely to suffer from chest infections such as *pneumonia* and *pleurisy*. Many of these lung diseases place an extra strain on the heart which can lead to *heart failure*. *Asthma* is another common condition that occurs in later life. Although a hereditary disease it is aggravated by smoking, infections and emotional upsets. The narrowing of the bronchial tubes is reversible in asthma, in contrast to the permanent lung damage caused by smoking.

Prevention

The cornerstone of preventing lung disease is *not to smoke*. It is never too late to stop, and although much of the damage to the lungs cannot be reversed, any further deterioration is halted. It is often when these diseases are advanced that they cause the most suffering, and quitting before this stage is reached allows smokers to remain in reasonably good health. The risk of heart disease and lung cancer is also reduced.

In older adults chest infections frequently complicate influenza. Therefore *vaccination*, particularly against influenza, is an important preventive measure. *Pollution*, *dust* and *fumes* are relatively minor factors contributing to lung disease, but they should also be avoided. Finally regular aerobic *exercise* is known to increase the efficiency of the heart and lungs.

ADULT IMMUNIZATION

Diseases such as polio, diphtheria and measles now rarely occur due to the success of childhood immunization. Adults, however, have been neglected and many remain unprotected against other preventable infectious diseases.

Almost every winter there is an outbreak of influenza ('the flu') with a number of people, particularly the frail and ill, developing pneumonia and some even dying. Immunization is an effective means of preventing influenza. It is advisable for people over sixty-five years of age and those who have heart, lung or other chronic diseases to receive the *flu injection*. Yearly vaccination is required as the virus is constantly changing, with a new strain appearing each winter. One injection provides sufficient protection and is administered in autumn to allow time for the body to develop immunity.

The effectiveness of vitamin C in combating flu and other respiratory infections continues to be vigorously debated.

Although unable to prevent these infections, vitamin C has been shown to reduce the effects of the cold virus and this has led to its widespread use as a 'natural' cold remedy. The dose taken is usually well above the normal body requirements, however, and side effects may be experienced (see pp 168–9).

A vaccine to protect against pneumonia is also available (pneumococcal vaccine). It is usually given only once but is reserved for the seriously ill and people who may die from pneumonia. Controversy surrounds whether it should be given to healthy older people.

Successful immunization programmes have resulted in complacency towards a number of serious infectious diseases. Tetanus germs are commonly present in the garden and can enter the body even through a small wound. Those who have never been vaccinated against tetanus and diphtheria require a course of three injections, but to maintain immunity only a single booster every ten years is needed. More frequent vaccination is required if an injury occurs. It is also important to keep an up-to-date and accurate record of all immunizations, not only during childhood but throughout adult life.

BOWEL DISORDERS

> To lower my cholesterol I am now eating fewer sweets and fatty foods but more fruit and vegetables. A pleasant surprise is that I am also no longer constipated, a problem that has troubled me for many years.
>
> Eleanor (63)

Diet is important in a number of bowel disorders. A western diet generally consists of many refined and processed foods which contribute to constipation, haemorrhoids and diverticular disease. These problems are not present in primitive societies where the food eaten contains more fibre.

Constipation is a common complaint in later life. The convenience of processed and packaged foods is preferred by many older people, particularly those who live alone and are not motivated to cook for themselves. These foods contain less roughage which is important for normal bowel function. Soft, less fibrous foods also tend to be eaten by people who have dental problems and experience difficulty chewing. In addition, drinking insufficient fluid contributes to constipation.

There is a widespread preoccupation with bowel regularity; consequently laxatives are frequently overused. These powerful drugs are best avoided, as they not only damage the muscles and nerves of the bowel, but can also become habit forming. Sometimes constipation is due to a disease and therefore any change in bowel habit warrants assessment by a doctor.

Haemorrhoids are the result of constipation and straining to pass hard motions. The veins in the 'back passage' swell like varicose veins causing discomfort and bleeding. As with constipation, bleeding from the bowel must be investigated as occasionally a cancer causes similar symptoms. The association between diet and bowel cancer is explained earlier in this chapter (p. 193).

A lack of dietary fibre produces motions that are difficult to propel through the large bowel. As the muscles in the bowel wall forcefully contract to move the motions, high pressures are produced which cause ballooning of the lining of the large bowel and the formation of little pockets. This condition is termed *diverticular disease*, or *diverticulitis* when these pockets become inflamed.

Irritable bowel syndrome is another common complaint, and fortunately it is not serious. It is the result of dietary as well as psychological factors, with the symptoms of pain and altered bowel habit easily confused with other diseases. Many of these problems can be avoided, or at the least alleviated, by eating a healthy balanced diet.

Prevention

Eating foods that contain fibre will maintain normal bowel function. Although unprocessed wheat bran is an excellent source of dietary fibre, it is not sufficient to simply sprinkle a teaspoon on cereal each morning and assume this will do the trick. Fibre should be obtained from a variety of sources including fruit, vegetables, legumes, wholemeal bread and wholegrain cereals. Cruciferous vegetables, as mentioned earlier, appear to have the added advantage of reducing the risk of bowel cancer. Some people feel bloated and suffer from 'wind' when fibre is introduced into their diet. This can usually be overcome by gradually increasing the amount of fibre eaten. Alternatively pharmaceutical preparations (bulking agents) are sometimes better tolerated than unprocessed bran. The fibre absorbs a lot of water which keeps the motions soft, bulky and easy to pass. Adequate amounts of fluid are therefore essential, and it is advisable to drink six to eight glasses of water each day.

A number of additional measures are required to prevent constipation. Bed rest, often associated with ill health, contributes to constipation and conversely exercise is beneficial in maintaining regularity. Some drugs, particularly codeine, antidepressants and antacids, can also cause constipation. When this occurs a doctor may be able to suggest an alternative treatment. Heeding 'the call of nature', rather than postponing it, will also allow a natural and regular bowel habit to develop.

URINARY INCONTINENCE

Whenever I played tennis urine would dribble onto my underwear. I was sure there was an odour and thought that my friends did not mention it because they were polite. Feeling too embarrassed to tell anybody I started giving weak excuses not to join them at tennis. I became quite depressed. Eventually I decided to seek help. The doctor suggested exercises to strengthen the muscles around the water passage and if this did not work an operation might be necessary. The exercises are simple and have been tremendously helpful. Thinking back I wish that I had done something earlier.

Lyn (60)

Urinary incontinence occurs when a person loses the ability to adequately control the passing of urine. This can range from a small leakage to a significant loss or flooding. It is estimated that 800 000 Australian adults suffer from this distressing problem, but due to embarrassment many conceal it even from close family and friends. Incontinence frequently causes them to feel ashamed, lose confidence and in extreme circumstances to become socially isolated. It can occur at any age but is more common in the elderly.

There has recently been a dramatic change in attitude towards incontinence. It is no longer accepted as a natural consequence of ageing and indeed many people benefit from treatment. The first step is for those affected not to feel embarrassed but to seek help. A thorough assessment can then be performed and an appropriate treatment plan suggested.

The sudden development of incontinence can usually be reversed by treating the cause. Urinary infections, constipation and drugs such as sedatives and 'water tablets' are common culprits. Sometimes pneumonia and other medical illnesses are responsible and the control of urine is regained when the person has recovered.

Incontinence that has been present for a long time can take a number of different forms. *Stress incontinence* is the leakage of a small amount of urine associated with coughing, sneezing or exercise. It is more common in women and is due to a weakening of the pelvic muscles which support the bladder, womb and bowel. These muscles have usually been stretched during childbirth and sag even more after menopause. Stress incontinence is worse in women who are overweight, suffer from constipation or have a 'smoker's cough', as these all place an extra strain on the pelvic muscles. Special exercises to strengthen these muscles are explained in Appendix 1. If practised regularly throughout life, pelvic exercises can prevent urinary incontinence.

The urge to pass urine can sometimes be so intense that the bladder empties before reaching a toilet. This is called *urge incontinence* and usually occurs in people with Parkinson's disease, dementia or those who have suffered a stroke. The sudden loss of urine is due to the involuntary contraction of the bladder muscles which have become unreliable and overactive. Bladder retraining has been shown to be an effective form of treatment for urge incontinence. Regular toileting, initially every two to three hours, helps regain continence, and as bladder control improves this time interval can be steadily increased. An alternative form of bladder training is beneficial if the bladder is small. It involves delaying or 'holding on' for a short period of time when there is the urge to urinate. This has the effect of enlarging the bladder and re-establishing control over the passing of urine. In addition, the common practice of reducing fluid intake is discouraged and people are advised to drink plenty of water. This additional fluid not only prevents dehydration and constipation, but also helps to stretch the bladder.

Overflow incontinence occurs when the bladder is unable to completely empty and therefore becomes too full, forcing urine to trickle out. This commonly occurs in men whose enlarged prostate blocks the flow of urine from the bladder. Treatment in this case involves a surgical operation to relieve the obstruction.

Obviously it is essential to be able to reach a toilet. Being bedridden or incapacitated alone can cause incontinence even though the urinary system is functioning normally. Improving mobility and providing a clear pathway to a close toilet will solve this problem.

Medication is available for incontinence, but this only has limited use as older people frequently experience undesirable side effects.

Although the majority of people benefit from treatment, a few may still remain incontinent. They can continue to be socially active by wearing special appliances or protective undergarments. Advice about incontinence can be obtained from local doctors or special 'continence clinics' whose staff are specifically trained to deal with this problem. In summary, measures which will help prevent incontinence include:

- Pelvic floor exercises (see Appendix 1);
- Avoid obesity;
- Regular bowel habit;
- Stop smoking; coughing aggravates stress incontinence;
- Drink adequate amounts of fluid;
- Avoid medication that causes incontinence (sedatives, fluid tablets).

PROSTATE DISEASE

The prostate gland lies immediately below a man's bladder and surrounds the tube that carries urine from the body. Enlargement of the prostate is common in later life and because of its position restricts the flow of urine. The extra growth can be due to a tumour which is usually benign. The operation to improve the flow of urine is performed through the penis by a special instrument that trims away the excess tissue. This operation does not affect sexual function, although sometimes semen can be diverted up to the bladder instead of being normally released from the penis.

There are no known causes for either the benign or cancerous enlargement of the prostate. Early detection is therefore the only effective preventive measure and involves a rectal examination. This test can be included as part of a routine yearly check up and is recommended for all men over fifty.

DEMENTIA

It was a shock when the doctor told us that Marge had Alzheimer's disease. I was totally unprepared as she had never been ill before. I always thought she would live longer than me and it took a long time to adjust. Although our friends congratulated me on how I coped, the most difficult part was not the house chores, but that I could no longer discuss things with her as we had always done. Looking back there was still a certain closeness and I am thankful that I was well enough to care for her.

Ted (75)

Dementia is essentially 'brain failure'. There are a number of different conditions that cause dementia, with Alzheimer's disease being the most common. They all result in a significant loss of mental abilities, which are severe enough to interfere with normal daily life.

Although the incidence of dementia increases with age, the majority of older people are not affected. At sixty-five years 5 per cent of people have dementia, with the number rising to 20 per cent in those aged eighty. It is the fourth most common cause of death after heart disease, cancer and strokes. As more people live longer, dementia is expected to become increasingly common. Not only are individual sufferers of the disease affected, but the burden is also shared by the families who care for them, as well as the wider community which has to provide appropriate facilities and nursing care.

Dementia is not a normal part of ageing. The derogatory term 'senile' is loosely applied to all changes in mental abilities that occur in later life. The word is negative and inaccurate. It does not differentiate between the devastating diseases that cause dementia and the minor normal effects of ageing.

Normal Forgetfulness

For many years I had noticed that I was forgetting names which I could previously remember. I had a fright the day after we moved from our home to a smaller unit and I could not remember the new phone number. Was this the beginning of senility? A visit to the doctor reassured me that this was normal and not the beginning of dementia.

Jim (68)

Forgetfulness occurs at all ages. While young people correctly dismiss it as an annoyance, for older adults it often triggers a fear that this may be the beginning of dementia. Minor memory difficulties do not interfere with everyday living and never progress to Alzheimer's disease. Some age related differences in mental function such as memory, learning and intelligence do occur, but these are not a simple matter of gradual decline, as will be discussed.

Forgetfulness is a common complaint in older people. Careful investigation has revealed that the three types of memory are not equally affected. *Immediate memory* is required to recall an address or phone number within a few seconds of seeing it. This form of memory is unaffected by age. If the address or phone number is left at home, trying to remember it some hours later relies on *short term memory*, which does decline with advancing years. Most older people are aware of this change and can compensate by keeping a list. *Long term memory*, recalling events that occured years ago, is not affected by age and many elderly people can accurately recall details of their youth.

Linked to memory is the ability to *learn*, and the saying that 'you can't teach an old dog new tricks' does not apply to older humans. The capacity to learn is maintained, although older adults tend to be slower, particularly if the information is unfamiliar. However, the loss of speed is compensated for in accuracy. The wisdom, knowledge and experience of age are advantages that can overcome caution and lack of speed.

Early studies into *intelligence* revealed a significant deterioration in later life. Subsequent investigation has found that most of the inequality between the generations is due to differences in background, education and opportunities rather than age. Vocabulary range, for example, tends to be wider in older adults, while the decline in other verbal skills is so slight as not to be noticeable. Non-verbal skills, required for domestic jobs and crafts, also decline. To detect these minor changes, sophisticated testing has to be performed, and therefore they do not present a problem in everyday life.

Many other factors affect intellectual function and age is often mistakenly blamed. Poor sight and hearing are common in later life and obviously affect an individual's ability to learn and understand. Ill health can directly interfere with the normal functioning of the brain causing confusion. In addition, isolation at home or in hospital deprives a person of normal mental stimulation.

Emotional worries, anxiety and depression can also influence concentration and memory. It is common to occasionally have trouble remembering a name when anxious or under pressure. Bereavement and grief normally take a long time to resolve and during this period of adjustment similar temporary changes may also be noticed. Sometimes these events can set up a vicious cycle, as the belief that mental functions are failing causes a further loss of confidence. Many 'problems' with memory, intelligence and learning are in fact normal minor alterations due to age which have been aggravated by the stresses encountered in later life. Age alone does not cause a significant decline in intelligence, memory or learning.

Improving Mental Function

An interesting and stimulating life is vital for those who wish to remain mentally alert. In later life this may require planning and effort as the previous challenges of work and parenting are no longer present. Interaction with other people, involvement in family affairs, belonging to organizations and participating in courses are some alternatives. Good health also improves mental performance, and exercise may even prevent a decline in mental as well as physical 'fitness'. Remaining relaxed is also important, as tension and pressure to remember quickly only increases anxiety which has a detrimental effect on memory. Concentrating is vital, particularly if loss of sight or hearing are problems.

There are a number of simple strategies to minimize being inconvenienced by these changes in memory. Developing organized habits, such as having a special place for keys, avoids the need to remember different locations each time. To memorize a person's name it is important to clearly hear the name, repeat it out loud and to mentally associate the name with something special, such as the occasion where the meeting occurred. Information can be learnt by using all the senses to imprint it in the mind; read, write and say out loud whatever has to be retained. Lists and a diary are other simple but practical memory aids that overcome normal forgetfulness.

The Causes of Dementia

The normal changes of ageing remain minor nuisances and never progress or interfere in daily life. Dementia is distinctly different. As dementia progresses significant events rather than small details are forgotten. For example, after meeting many new friends at a party it would not be unusual to have difficulty remembering some of their names. A person with dementia would be unable even to recall being at the party. In addition to memory loss, dementia interferes with other functions of the brain such as thinking and reasoning. Language, mood and behaviour are also affected. Frequently the problem becomes so disabling that the demented person is not capable of managing his or her own life. At this stage considerable support from other people is required.

Alzheimer's disease and multiple strokes (multi-infarct dementia) are the most common causes of dementia. They are both irreversible. A number of other conditions have symptoms that can easily be confused with dementia but which can be reversed. These include medical illnesses such as thyroid disease and infections. Depression also frequently mimics dementia. It is crucial, therefore, that people suspected of suffering from dementia undergo a thorough examination.

TABLE 7.2 The main causes of dementia

Cause	%
Alzheimer's disease	50%
Multi-infarct dementia	20%
Reversible causes (e.g. depression, medical illnesses)	20%
Others (many are rare)	10%

Alzheimer's Disease

This devastating disease is due to the brain degenerating in a characteristic way. It begins insidiously with sufferers forgetting recent events but still remembering the past. They seem more apathetic and often become anxious or depressed in the early stages of the illness as they recognize that there is a problem. Over the years Alzheimer's disease progresses relentlessly, resulting in a progressive loss of intellectual abilities. Those affected become increasingly confused and can forget to do even simple tasks such as washing and turning off the gas. Important documents are lost, the same questions repeatedly asked and the ability to make decisions impaired. They become lost even in familiar surroundings and may not even know the date or year. Their command of language can also deteriorate, from having trouble finding the right words to the stage of no longer being able to speak. Behavioural problems and changes in mood can be the most difficult for their family to cope with. Sadly, in the advanced stages of the illness, victims of Alzheimer's disease may no longer recognize their own spouse and children. Help is generally required for toileting, dressing and feeding, and institutional care may be required.

The cause of Alzheimer's disease remains a mystery. Microscopic examination of the brain reveals plaques and tangles of nerves. Abnormal protein is also present and the chemicals involved in communication between nerve cells are reduced. Viruses and aluminium are two suggested causes but the evidence implicating them is not impressive.

Currently there is a lot of interest in the role of genetics in the development of Alzheimer's disease. It appears that family members have only a slightly increased risk of developing the disease.

There are no memory enhancing drugs and Alzheimer's disease cannot be cured. Treatment is aimed at ensuring that these people are comfortable and feel loved. The present approach is to maximize their remaining mental function by providing a stimulating but simple environment which encourages them to remain well-orientated. There is further research being done into the disease and in time more satisfactory forms of treatment may become available.

Multi-infarct Dementia

Multi-infarct dementia is caused by a series of small strokes. Individually each stroke is minor but as the damage accumulates many functions of the brain are affected. The symptoms of multi-infarct dementia are similar to those of Alzheimer's disease.

Prevention of Dementia

The prevention of dementia depends on its cause. Those that are reversible and masquerade as dementia can usually be cured, and a number even prevented. Depression in later life can easily be mistaken for dementia and the term 'pseudo-dementia' is often used for this. Depressed people are preoccupied with their own thoughts and problems. They are unable to concentrate and may neglect other aspects of their life. With appropriate treatment the depression will resolve, allowing normal memory and intellectual function to return.

The brain is also very sensitive to change. A decrease in the amount of oxygen due to heart or lung disease can result in confusion. Treatment of these medical conditions will restore normal thought processes. Similarly alcohol and drugs, particularly 'nerve tablets', can adversely affect the brain. These reversible conditions should always be considered as possible causes of dementia-like symptoms. If they are not detected the person may be incorrectly labelled as demented.

Appropriate assessment and treatment is essential to avoid these pitfalls.

Multi-infarct dementia, although irreversible once it has developed, can be avoided by implementing the preventive measures previously described for the more usual forms of stroke (pp. 185–6). This involves correcting risk factors such as high blood pressure, smoking and diabetes. Warning strokes [TIA] should not be ignored as aspirin can prevent more serious strokes.

Alzheimer's disease remains the most common cause of dementia but unfortunately it cannot be prevented. Certain factors may accelerate the decline in mental function. This deterioration can be slowed by allowing those with Alzheimer's disease to continue interacting with other people, as well as attending to sight and hearing problems which isolate them from the outside world. Other physical illnesses should be treated and care taken when prescribing drugs that affect the brain. As the disease itself cannot be significantly influenced, the quality of life for the sufferers of Alzheimer's disease is largely determined by the quality of the care they receive. The emphasis should therefore also focus on preventing unnecessary strain on caregivers. They commonly carry the burden of physical, emotional and financial hardship alone, and their job is difficult, exhausting and often thankless. For a more detailed discussion of the problems which may be encountered by caregivers, and how to avoid or minimize these, turn to pages 38–41.

The Alzheimer's Disease and Related Disorders Society (ADARDS), was formed to meet the needs of both sufferers of Alzheimer's disease and their carers. It provides information, advice and offers practical suggestions on ways of coping with a variety of problems that are commonly encountered. Support groups are one of the important functions of ADARDS. Feelings of hopelessness, frustration, anger and guilt are common emotions experienced by caregivers. Being able to express and discuss these feelings with people who are not judgemental and have overcome similar difficulties is extremely beneficial. Preventing these problems from over-whelming the caregiver will improve the quality of life for both the carers and sufferers of Alzheimer's disease.

PARKINSON'S DISEASE

Parkinson's disease is a chronic neurological disorder which usually does not occur before fifty-five years of age. It is characterized by tremor, muscle stiffness and slow movements, which interfere with walking and speech. Effective medication is now available, allowing many people who have Parkinson's disease to remain active and enjoy a good quality of life.

Degeneration of special cells in the base of the brain and depletion of the important chemicals they produce leads to Parkinson's disease. It is believed environmental factors initiate these changes but the exact cause remains unknown. Prevention therefore remains focused on minimizing disability rather than on preventing the disease. Medication, physiotherapy and emotional support from family and friends enables those with Parkinson's disease to lead an independent, full and useful life for many years.

DEPRESSION

For a long time after Helen died I felt depressed and lonely. Feeling this way would not change anything and I realized that there was still a lot to live for. I was missing out on enjoying my children and grandchildren, and started visiting them regularly. I began to go out and meet people. I joined a walking club. As well as feeling fitter I am more satisfied with my life. Surprisingly I have become involved with a lady and her friendship has been most comforting.

Joe (75)

Depression is a common human emotion and normal in circumstances such as bereavement. Feeling depressed can range from being unhappy or down, through to a severe and incapacitating depressive illness. Feelings of depression in later life are usually transient episodes of sadness that eventually resolve by themselves. However, severe depression does occur and should not be ignored as it will improve with appropriate treatment.

There are two types of depression. *Endogenous* depression may develop without any obvious reason, while *reactive* depression is usually the result of external factors such as stressful events and ill health. Later life is punctuated by a number of losses that can contribute to depression. It is common for older people to suffer the loss of someone they love, with feelings of profound sadness being a normal part of grief. It is also a time of transition with retirement, and the associated loss of status.

Ill health can have a dramatic impact on the way a person feels. The discomfort of chronic pain is demoralizing and a constant reminder of illness. Disability due to a stroke, fractured hip or impaired sight and hearing can cause a loss of independence leading to isolation and loneliness. Even certain medications used in the treatment of these illnesses can themselves cause depression.

Older people are generally not valued by society and this too contributes to a lowering of self-esteem. Despite these adversities, however, the majority of older people are able to cope. They are well-adjusted and satisfied with their lives. Depression tends to occur only in those who are vulnerable, rather than in everyone who is confronted by stress or a loss.

Depressive illness can manifest itself in a variety of ways. People who are depressed often feel miserable and worthless. They lack confidence and view with pessimism any problems that arise. Sleep disturbances and crying are also common. Overwhelmed by feelings of remorse there is a risk that they will withdraw from social activities and friendships, and this loneliness compounds the problem. Unfortunately many older people accept the tiredness and lassitude of depression as a normal part of ageing. Frequently a variety of physical symptoms will mask depression. Pain, palpitations and weight loss are often the body's way of signalling that a person is emotionally upset. Those who are depressed dwell on their problems and this may interfere with concentration and memory (pseudodementia). The ultimate risk in depression is the possibility of suicide. Surprisingly, research has shown that it is ill elderly men living alone who have the highest rate of suicide, rather than the more publicized younger generation. People suspected of being depressed should always seek professional help, as most will improve with treatment.

Prevention

At present endogenous depression cannot be prevented as its cause remains unknown. People may be able to avoid reactive depression, however, by reducing the amount of stress induced by lifetime events such as retirement and moving from the family home. Planning for retirement will buffer its impact on daily life. When moving to different accommodation the emotional effects should also be considered, not simply the physical advantages that may be gained. Many similar problems can be averted by careful consideration after discussing the various options with family and friends. While feeling depressed following a crisis or bereavement, it is advisable not to make important decisions.

Individuals can themselves avoid feeling sad by positive thinking. Remembering past achievements and enjoyable experiences reinforces self-worth. This will often bolster a person's confidence in their ability to overcome the obstacles that still confront them. Accepting that some events will be distressing, but knowing there is always a solution, prevents self-pity.

A close friend or confidante can be invaluable. During a crisis the support of a trusted friend is a help in coping with adverse circumstances. This may involve having someone who will listen and discuss a problem, or on other occasions providing more practical assistance. A confiding and intimate relationship improves morale and has a positive effect on mental health.

Later life can also be a time to start new interests and pleasures that previously were impossible due to other commitments. These can result in new friendships forming. Participation in clubs, sporting groups or simply continuing to meet old friends are all valuable social activities. They should not be restricted to people of a similar age, as a broad range of friends adds variety and interest. Many older people find the bonds with their grandchildren to be special and uniquely rewarding. Involvement with other people promotes feelings of self-worth and prevents loneliness.

Ill health and depression are closely linked. A healthy lifestyle, as detailed in earlier chapters, will prevent many diseases from developing. Those people who become ill will be less apprehensive if the disease and its treatment are explained. It is important to understand and be involved in these medical decisions. It is hardly surprising that disability and loss of independence also cause depression. This can often be alleviated by treatment and supplying appropriate aids. For example, a person who is unable to climb stairs will no longer be housebound when a ramp or handrail is fitted. If these measures are implemented early, depression will be prevented. Finally drugs that are known to cause depression should be avoided. These include sedatives and some tablets used to treat high blood pressure.

Some elderly people silently suffer from depression. It is often accepted by their friends and relatives as normal or part of ageing. If depression is suspected, seeking professional help and treatment will usually bring relief.

SLEEPLESSNESS

Now that I have finally stopped taking sleeping tablets I feel less 'groggy' in the morning and more in control of my life. I sleep less than before but it seems to be enough.

Beryl (63)

Sleeplessness can be a distressing problem. There is a great deal of individual variation in the amount of sleep required, and feeling rested rather than counting the hours spent in bed or asleep is the best guide to adequate sleep. Many older people report problems with sleeping, but often these are normal changes that occur with age.

Those in later life should not expect to have eight hours of uninterrupted sleep as they did in their youth. Most older people require less sleep, with five to six hours sometimes being sufficient. Other normal changes include a delay in falling asleep and frequent awakenings throughout the night. The result is a fragmented light sleep. These differences are not dangerous and seldom interfere with daytime activities. They certainly do not indicate a need for sleeping tablets. After retirement there is a tendency to nap during the day and this can also adversely affect sleeping at night. Older adults should adjust their sleeping habits to fit with these normal ageing changes by spending less time in bed.

Other factors, of which stress is the most common, can interfere with sleep. It is preferable to settle arguments and resolve problems before going to bed. If this cannot be done then relaxation exercises may be beneficial in relieving anxiety and tension. Depression is another emotional complaint which typically causes early morning waking. Arthritic pain, breathlessness from heart or lung disorders and waking to pass urine also disturb sleep. Many of these medical and emotional problems can be improved by appropriate treatment.

Some people stop breathing for short periods of time while asleep. This condition is called *sleep apnea*; sleep is disturbed which results in feeling tired and lethargic during the day. Sleep apnea is associated with snoring and may contribute to high blood pressure. People who have this condition benefit from losing weight, avoiding sedatives including alcohol and not sleeping on their back. If these simple measures are unsuccessful then medical advice should be sought.

Unfortunately medication is often the first and only option considered for improving sleep. Many problems are associated with sleeping tablets of which addiction is the most serious. Except in rare circumstances these drugs should not be used for longer than two weeks. The sleep they induce is less restful and of a poorer quality. In addition a hangover and drowsiness may be experienced the next day.

People who have been taking sleeping tablets for a long period of time and wish to stop should consult their doctor for advice. Being addictive these drugs must be reduced gradually as rebound insomnia (a significant worsening of sleep disturbances) and other withdrawal problems can occur.

Prevention

Good sleeping habits promote a restful and natural sleep without drugs. Regular exercise and enjoyable activities usually ensure a sounder sleep. A daytime nap can disrupt sleep at night and should therefore be avoided. Waking at the same time each day allows the body's own internal clock to be set, which encourages a regular sleeping pattern.

A number of socially accepted drugs affect sleep. The stimulating effect of caffeine in coffee, tea, chocolate and cola drinks is well known, and drinking these in the evening tends to keep people awake. It is also advisable to limit coffee to no more three cups a day. Similarly, the nicotine in cigarettes is a stimulant. Although an alcoholic drink as a 'nightcap' helps a person to fall asleep, the effects of withdrawal can cause arousal and waking some hours later. There is also a danger of alcohol addiction if the sleeping problems continue; it is therefore not a cure for insomnia.

A regular routine facilitates sleep. This can begin with winding down before going to bed. Restful music, reading or special relaxation techniques are some suggestions. The time honoured habit of a warm bath and glass of milk is also effective in promoting sleep. Rather than going to bed at a specific time and remaining awake for hours it is preferable to go to sleep when feeling pleasantly tired. Bed should be reserved for sleep and sex, with other activities such as watching television and eating performed in more appropriate places. A comfortable, quiet and dark room will also ensure a sounder sleep. Finally, knowing that most older people sleep lightly and for fewer hours will prevent unnecessary concern about altered sleep patterns in later life.

SIGHT AND HEARING

Sight and hearing are special senses that keep people informed about the world around them. Sight is necessary for many aspects of daily living including reading and driving. Hearing is important as it maintains communication and contact with other people. The ability to remain active, independent and enjoy a good quality of life is significantly influenced by the function of these senses.

Sight

Because my mother had glaucoma I have always arranged to have my eyes checked regularly. It has paid off as the specialist found the same problem. He has reassured me that treatment will reduce the pressure in the eye and my sight will remain normal.

Joan (67)

Fortunately the majority of older people maintain reasonably good sight which enables them to continue their normal work and pursue a variety of personal interests. It is important to differentiate between poor vision due to the normal effects of ageing and the loss of vision due to diseases such as cataracts and glaucoma.

Reading and other activities that require close vision often become more difficult in later life. This decline in sight is due to ageing of the lens in the eye, which is less able to change shape and focus on nearby objects. This can always be corrected by wearing glasses as the eyes are still healthy.

Diseases and not age cause permanent visual problems that interfere with daily living. Cataracts, glaucoma, senile macular degeneration and diabetes are common causes of poor vision. Cataracts are due to the lens of the eye becoming cloudy, and this is frequently accepted by older people as due to ageing. However when the cataract significantly interferes with normal living sight can be restored by surgically removing the damaged lens and implanting an artificial one.

Eye damage caused by glaucoma is more insidious and frequently not noticed until there has been an irreversible loss of vision. Glaucoma is due to increased pressure within the eye, and is able to be measured. Often there are no symptoms, making routine testing necessary. This is particularly important in relatives of people who have this problem. Glaucoma can usually be successfully treated, therefore early detection and treatment will prevent loss of vision.

Damage to the light sensitive lining of the eye, the retina, causes a loss of sight that is almost always permanent. Senile macular degeneration and diabetes are the two most common disorders that affect the retina. Senile macular degeneration damages the area of the retina that is concerned with central vision (called the macula). This results in difficulty seeing straight ahead which is important for reading and driving. There is no cure for senile macular degeneration although some evidence suggests that laser treatment may be beneficial if this problem is detected early. The outlook for preventing eye problems caused by diabetes is more optimistic as good control of diabetes can prevent these complications. It has also been shown that laser treatment in the early stages will stop further damage to the retina.

Diabetics require regular eye examinations to detect early charges.

Prevention

A routine *health check-up* will usually incorporate measuring blood pressure and testing for diabetes, the two medical conditions which can affect vision. In addition, *specialist examination* of the eyes by an optometrist or ophthalmologist should be done every two years and more frequently if a problem such as diabetes is present. Unfortunately many causes of blindness cannot be cured and therefore *early detection* is vital. Glaucoma and diabetes can be successfully treated in the early stages. It is also important for people to *immediately report eye symptoms* such as pain or loss of vision to their doctor. These measures will reduce the number of serious eye problems. Where treatment is unsuccessful, they can obtain advice and support from the Blind Institutes in each state, which will enable them to remain informed, active and independent members of the community.

Hearing

The stigma of wearing a hearing aid contrasts with the general acceptance of eye glasses and reflects the differences in attitude towards impaired sight and hearing. There is generally less sympathy for deaf people than for those who have poor sight. Difficulty in hearing can provoke annoyance and frustration in other people, who often attribute misunderstandings to foolishness or stupidity rather than simply an inability to hear. This prejudice is unfortunate as some degree of hearing impairment is present in one third of people over sixty-five years of age.

Hearing is important in communicating with other people and plays a central role in maintaining friendships and socialising. Hearing impairment can result in depression, loss of confidence, withdrawal and social isolation. Paranoia may even occur if sufficient suspicion is aroused in a deaf person who cannot understand or participate in conversations.

Hearing loss is due to a variety of causes. Wax in the ear is a simple problem to rectify. A number of other conditions, such as infections or fluid in the middle ear, can be effectively treated with medication. An overgrowth of bone (oto-sclerosis) can also occur, with hearing being restored by an operation. Some very powerful antibiotics, which are only used to treat serious infections, can permanently damage the ear and reduce hearing. Even drugs such as aspirin can cause hearing problems which fortunately are reversed when the aspirin is stopped.

Most hearing loss in later life is due to biological ageing of the hearing apparatus (presbycusis). It develops slowly over many years, and the change may be so gradual that a person is unaware of the deterioration. Exposure to excessive noise contributes to this loss. The high frequency sounds like 's, t, sh and ch' are most difficult for older people to hear, therefore they miss out on parts of words or sentences as sounds become indistinct and muffled. This makes conversation more difficult to follow.

Prevention

For the one older person in three who suffers from hearing loss, age itself is believed to be the most common cause. It is therefore unavoidable. The aim of prevention is to minimize the amount of disability that may be caused by poor hearing, as well as improving communication with other people.

It is not unusual for older adults to be unaware that their hearing is reduced. They may continue to deny having difficulty even when it is brought to their attention. The first step then, is to recognize and admit that a problem exists. Appropriate advice can then be sought and solutions found. Hearing aids, amplification of the telephone and a flashing light to signal that the door bell has been rung are effective ways of overcoming hearing loss and maintaining a normal life.

Hearing aids are not perfect in restoring age related deafness but they will maximize the remaining hearing. Simply fitting a hearing aid is not sufficient. Each person should be individually instructed in how the aid can best be used, and family and friends should learn ways they can improve their communication with the deaf person.

At all ages it is essential to protect hearing from loud noise. Work is where most people are exposed to unacceptably loud sounds, but even in retirement a noisy lawn mower can contribute to a further loss of hearing. Wearing special ear plugs or muffs will prevent this damage. Maintaining good hearing enables continued involvement in social activities and improves communication with other people. Deaf people may be 'cut off' from good quality communication, which results in a loss of self-esteem. Below are listed some ways to improve communication with a person who is unable to hear well:

- speak clearly;
- speak loudly but do not shout;
- stand where the person listening can see you clearly;
- don't speak while eating or chewing and avoid covering your mouth;
- use other means to help get the message across:
  — touch the person to attract their attention
  — use facial expressions and hand gestures
  — write messages
- reduce background noise — turn off the television and radio;
- rephrase misunderstood sentences rather than simply repeating them;
- treat deaf people with dignity and respect;
- do not be embarrassed to tell people about your hearing problem.

DENTAL CARE

Dental problems can cause poor nutrition in the elderly because the teeth are necessary for chewing. Less obvious is the importance of teeth in facial appearance and speech, both of which affect self-esteem. Many older people incorrectly accept the loss of their teeth as an inevitable part of ageing. Tooth decay and gum disease, not age, are the major causes of tooth loss. Both these conditions are due to plaque which is a sticky film on the teeth and gums that contains damaging bacteria. If not removed, the plaque causes tooth decay and infected bleeding gums. Gum disease can spread to the structures holding the tooth, eventually leading to the tooth being lost. Good oral hygiene will prevent these problems.

Correct dental care aims to prevent the build-up of plaque on teeth and gums. Sugar allows the harmful bacteria to multiply and therefore snacks, particularly of sweet sticky foods, should be avoided. For strong healthy teeth it is important to eat a balanced diet containing protein, milk products, fruit and vegetables. Flouride in water is also believed to strengthen an older person's teeth against decay.

Brushing teeth at least twice daily, preferably after eating, is an essential part of dental hygiene. It not only cleans the teeth but also massages the gums. Dentists are best qualified to demonstrate the correct brushing technique, and will usually advise that a soft bristle toothbrush and flouride toothpaste be used. Dental floss cleans between the teeth where the toothbrush cannot reach and supplements brushing. If bleeding or pain occurs while brushing and flossing it is advisable to see a dentist.

Regular twice yearly dental check ups are necessary throughout life. In addition to cleaning and removing plaque a dentist will treat any tooth or gum problem so that the maximum number of teeth are retained. It is also important to check for mouth cancer. Red or white patches in the mouth or a sore that does not heal may be a cancer. Smoking and alcohol contribute to mouth cancer.

Dentures require proper care to maintain a fresh and healthy mouth. They must be brushed and washed daily to remove the plaque. At night take out the dentures and soak them in water. It is also advisable to rinse the mouth with warm salt water after meals. Regular visits to the dentist should continue despite the absence of teeth. This is to check that the denture fits correctly and to examine the mouth for cancer. Those who continue to care for their teeth will be rewarded with better nutrition and an attractive smile.

SKIN AGEING

For years I sat in the sun to get a tan which I believed helped me look attractive. Now at 60 I spend a lot of time and money on cosmetics to conceal the damage caused by the sun!

Alice (60)

Skin changes are the most visible sign of ageing. Interestingly there is evidence of a correlation between external physical changes as seen in the skin, and biological ageing of the body's internal organs. Those who appear younger than their years will often feel, behave and function at a younger age. Physical appearance is also important psychologically. If people are well-groomed and have cared for themselves, it is likely they will feel more confident and have a high self-esteem.

An important part of remaining healthy involves proper skin care. With the passing of years the skin loses its elasticity and becomes dry, rough and wrinkled. Some of these changes are an inevitable part of ageing, but others are due to environmental factors. Exposure to the wind and sun, poor nutrition and smoking all accelerate the ageing of skin.

Prevention

Sun damage is the most important preventable factor and has earned the title 'photoageing'. This is separate from natural ageing and causes increased wrinkling, yellowing and dryness of the skin which gives it a leathery look. Most people are aware of the relationship between skin cancer and exposure to the sun. The advice is the same for preventing ageing of the skin due to the harmful rays of the sun. Wearing a hat and protective clothing, applying sunscreens and avoiding the sun in the middle of the day (11 am–3 pm summer time) are precautions that prevent both cancer and ageing of the skin. It is never too late to implement these measures, as they not only prevent further damage but there is also evidence that the skin can repair itself. Some cosmetic companies have recognized the importance of protection from the sun and include a sunscreen as an ingredient in their cosmetic preparations. Fortunately the idea that a tan indicates good health is changing, and the reality that it is a sign of skin damage is more widely known.

To minimize drying of the skin excessive amounts of soap should not be used. These remove the skin's natural oils which are only slowly replaced in older people by fewer and less efficient sebaceous(oil) glands. Similarly, excessive use of toners and cleansers can dry the skin. Regular application of a moisturiser prevents this drying by supplementing the skin's natural oils and reducing the loss of water. The result is skin which feels smooth and looks less wrinkled.

Although female hormones are usually prescribed for the relief of menopausal problems such as hot flushes and osteoporosis, they also have a beneficial effect on skin, giving it a more youthful appearance.

Vitamin-A has long been known to be important in maintaining healthy skin. The main dietary sources of vitamin A, or its derivative beta-carotene, are in the yellow-orange fruit and vegetables, for example carrots. It has also recently been discovered that when applied to the skin, a synthetic derivative of vitamin A (tretinoin cream marketed as Retin-A), can reduce the skin wrinkles due to photoageing. Tretinoin cream had been used successfully for many years to treat acne, until it was incidentally noted that the skin of older people became smoother and less wrinkled. This medication is however not a miracle cure or a fountain of youth for ageing skin. It takes time for the full benefits to be noticed, with the improvement being only modest. The response to tretinoin cream also varies; the most benefit is gained by those with a fair complexion, while for many other individuals the changes are minimal. The question of how long the benefits will last after ceasing treatment remains unanswered. Adverse reactions have been reported and include dryness, redness, scaling and itch. More work needs to be done before this cream or other derivatives of vitamin A are given unqualified endorsement, but to date the findings have been exciting.

Cosmetic surgery is another alternative that is readily available and popular with certain sections of the community. The final choice for surgery rests with the individual after evaluating the realistic benefits against the discomfort and risk of surgery.

A smile is still the best anti-ageing skin cosmetic.

TABLE 7.3 Minimising skin ageing

Avoid sun exposure

- avoid the midday sun (11 am–3 pm summer time);
- wear a hat and protective clothing; sit in the shade;
- use sunscreens; apply to skin that cannot be naturally protected;
- the higher the Sun Protection Factor number the greater the protection from the damaging radiation of the sun — SPF 15+ gives maximum protection;
- apply sunscreens at least half an hour before exposure;
- some cosmetics contain sunscreens but check the sun protection factor number.

Eat a balanced diet

- foods containing vitamin A.

Do not smoke

- smoking reduces the blood flow and the nourishment to the skin.

Minimize exposure to the elements

- avoid sun and wind in summer;
- avoid dry heat in winter.

Avoid excessive use of soap (bath oils are an alternative).

Apply moisturizers regularly.

Medications

- female hormone replacement in post-menopausal women;
- Tretinoin cream, researching the possibility that this may rejuvenate skin.

APPENDIX 1
PELVIC MUSCLE
EXERCISES

The muscles around the pelvis (pelvic muscles) are very important in supporting the bladder, urethra, vagina and rectum. Following childbirth or with advancing age, these muscles may weaken. They can be strengthened by regularly practising pelvic muscle exercises. If practised throughout life, these exercises will reduce the chances of becoming incontinent. These exercises are described below. A physiotherapist may be able to assist in assessing and teaching them.

Stage One

In order to identify the correct muscles to exercise, do the following exercises during the first week:

1. To identify the muscles around the back passage (rectum), sit or stand comfortably and imagine that you are trying to control diarrhoea by consciously tightening the ring of muscles around the back passage. Hold this squeeze for four seconds each time.
2. Go to the toilet and commence passing urine. Now try to stop the flow of urine midstream. Once this is done recommence voiding until the bladder is emptied. The muscles used to slow or stop the flow of urine are the front pelvic muscles which help control the bladder.
3. Some women find they can identify the correct pelvic muscles by inserting a finger into the vagina, then squeezing the finger by contracting the pelvic muscles. If the finger cannot be felt, then probably the wrong muscles are being exercised or the muscles are still very weak. Do not give up but proceed to stage two exercises.

Note

- Do not bear down as if trying to pass a bowel motion (or as a woman would do during childbirth). This strengthens the wrong muscles and may make incontinence worse!

Stage Two

Now that the correct muscles have been identified, the following pelvic exercises should be performed every day. They should *not* be done while passing urine.

1. While sitting or standing with thighs slightly apart, contract the muscles around the back passage then hold the front muscles around the vagina. Hold this contraction while slowing counting to five. Now relax the muscles. Repeat this four more times. Try to be aware of the squeezing and lifting sensation in the pelvis that frequently occurs when these exercises are done correctly.
2. While sitting or standing, tighten the muscles around the front and back passages together. Hold the contraction for just one second and relax. Repeat this exercise five times in quick succession.

Note

- These 'slow and quick' exercises are important to strengthen the pelvic muscles properly.
- At stage two, it is not appropriate to do the stage one exercise of stopping the urine each time urine is passed at the toilet. This is only a preliminary exercise.
- These exercises should be done every hour but certainly *not less than four times each day*.
- With practice, the exercises described should be quite easy to master and they can be carried out at any time — while waiting for a bus, watching television or standing at the sink. There is no need to interrupt the daily routine.
- Once every week or so it is important to return to stage one for a quick check that the correct muscles are being used.
- While these exercises are particularly useful for women, they may also be helpful for men, especially those suffering from dribbling or urgency.

APPENDIX 2
USEFUL ADDRESSES

General Advice

National
Australian Council on the
Ageing
3rd floor, 464 St Kilda Road
Melbourne 3004
Tel: 03 820 2655

Australian Capital Territory
ACT Council on the Ageing
Hughes Community Centre
Hughes 2605
Tel: 06 282 3777

Canberra Pensioners Social
and Recreational Club
Childers Street
Canberra 2600
Tel: 06 247 3797

Commonwealth Office for the
Aged
Department of Community
Services and Health
GPO Box 9848
Woden 2606
Tel: 062 89 5246

New South Wales
NSW Council on the Ageing
34 Argyle Place
Sydney 2000
Tel: 02 247 4857

Australian Pensioners And
Superannuants Federation
405 Sussex Street
Sydney 2000
Tel: 02 281 5951, 02 281 1811

NSW Office for Ageing
State Office Block
74 Phillip Street
Sydney 2000
Tel: 02 228 4250

Older Women's Network
87 Lower Fort Street
Millers Point 2000
Tel: 02 247 7046

Northern Territory
NT Council on the Ageing
PO Box 2476
Darwin 0801
Tel: 089 41 1173

Darwin Pensioners and Senior
Citizens Association Inc
PO Box 852
Darwin 0801
Tel: 089 81 9691

Queensland
Queensland Council on the
Ageing
Sir Leslie Wilson Youth Centre
10th Avenue

Windsor 4030
Tel: 07 857 6877

Australian Pensioners and
Superannuants League
Queensland Inc
PO Box 141
West End 4101
Tel: 07 844 5878

Department of Family Services
GPO Box 806
Brisbane 4001
Tel: 07 224 2111

Later Years Ltd
168 Edward Street
Brisbane 4001
Tel: 07 221 2977, 211 2230

South Australia
SA Council on the Ageing
45 Flinders Street
Adelaide 5000
Tel: 08 232 0422

Voice Of The Elderly (VOTE)
24 Grace Road
Darlington 5047
Tel: 08 296 3454

Office of the Commissioner
for the Aged
PO Box 70
Rundle Mall
Adelaide 5000
Tel: 08 226 7050

Tasmania
Tasmanian Council on the
Ageing
2 St Johns Avenue
New Town 7008
Tel: 002 28 1897

Tasmanian Pensioners' Union
156 Elizabeth Street
Hobart 7000
Tel: 002 34 8526

Department of Health Services
34 Davey Street
Hobart 7000
Tel: 002 30 8011

Victoria
Victorian Council on the
Ageing
126 Wellington Parade
Melbourne 3002
Tel: 03 416 0822

The Combined Pensioners'
Association of Victoria
54 Victoria Street
Carlton 3053
Tel: 03 662 3971

Older Persons' Planning Office
500 Bourke Street
Melbourne 3000
Tel: 03 602 0536

Older Persons' Action Centre
247 Flinders Lane
Melbourne 3000
Tel: 03 650 4709

Western Australia
Council on the Ageing (WA)
Inc
11 Freedman Road
Mount Lawley 6050
Tel: 09 272 2133

Pensioners' Action Group —
WA Inc
79 Stirling Street
Perth 6000
Tel: 09 220 0656

Bureau for the Aged
35 Haveloch Street
West Perth 6005
Tel: 09 30 8011

Retirement

Australian Capital Territory
National Clearing House on
Pensioner Investments
Suite 4, Kingston House
86 Giles Street
Kingston 2604
Tel: 06 239 6722, 008 02110

New South Wales
Australian Retired Persons
Association
60–70 Elizabeth Street
Sydney 2000
Tel: 02 233 6163

Australian Information
Services for Pensioners
Level 3A, 405 Sussex Street
Sydney 2000
Tel: 02 281 4566

Queensland
Australian Retired Persons
Association
Penny's Building
210 Queen Street
Brisbane 4000
Tel: 07 221 6920

South Australia
Australian Retired Persons
Association
Satfac House
151 South Terrace
Adelaide 5000
Tel: 08 231 0171

Tasmania
Australian Retired Persons
Association
PO Box 36
Rosny Park 7108
Tel: 002 43 8714

Victoria
Australian Retired Persons
Association
150 Queens Street
Melbourne 3000
Tel: 03 670 6275

Victorian Retirement
Advisory Association
258 Bourke Street
Melbourne 3000
Tel: 03 663 6269

The Early Planning and
Retirement Association
449 Swantson Street
Melbourne 3000
Tel: 03 663 3235

Women's Retirement
Association Inc
Second Floor, Bible House
341 Flinders Lane
Melbourne 3000
Tel: 03 337 8247

Over Fifties Association of
Victoria
358 Lonsdale Street
Melbourne 3000
Tel: 03 670 6275

Don't Overlook Mature
Expertise (DOME)
370 Camberwell Road
Camberwell
Tel: 03 882 4488

Retired Persons Federation of
Australia
State Bank Building
258 Little Bourke Street
Melbourne 3000
Tel: 03 663 3204

Western Australia
Australian Retired Persons
Association
McNess Hall
8/14 Pier Street
Perth 6000
Tel: 09 325 7409

Housing

Victoria
Abbeyfield Societies
141A Queens Parade
Clifton Hill
Melbourne 3068
Tel: 03 481 4400

Grandparenthood

Victoria
Foster Grandparents
Ross House
247 Flinders Lane
Melbourne 3000
Tel: 03 650 7216

Grandparents Support Group
C/- Leila Friedman
2/29 Gnarwyn Road
Carnegie 3163
Tel: 03 568 3306

Companionship

New South Wales
Do Care Programs
210 Pitt Street

Sydney 3000
Tel: 02 267 8741

South Australia
Do Care Programs
43 Franklin Street
Adelaide 5000
Tel: 08 212 2599

Victoria
Do Care Programs
148 Lonsdale Street
Melbourne 3000
Tel: 03 662 2044

Carers

Australian Capital Territory
ACT Carers' Group
Hughes Community Centre
Wisdom Street
Hughes 2605
Tel: 06 282 3777

New South Wales
Carers' Association of NSW
Inc.
PO Box 84
Darlinghurst 2010
Tel: 02 361 6353

Victoria
Caring for Family Caregivers
Australia
109 Drummond Street
Carlton 3053
Tel: 03 663 2855

Queensland
Queensland Council of Carers
15 Abbott Street
Camp Hill 4152
Tel: 07 843 1401

South Australia
South Australia Carers'
Association
23 Coglin Street
Adelaide 5000
Tel: 08 212 2057

Western Australia
Western Australia Carers'
Council
c/o 5 Albion Street
Craigie 6025

Grief

Australian Capital Territory
Solace Association Inc
Tel: 062 31 8802

New South Wales
National Association for Loss
and Grief
PO Box 79
Turramurra 2074
Tel: 02 988 3376

Solace Association Inc
Tel: 02 519 2820

Queensland
National Association for Loss
and Grief
302 Bennetts Road
Norman Park 4170
Tel: 07 881 1505

South Australia
National Association for Loss
and Grief
63 Clairville Road
Campbelltown 5074
Tel: 08 336 2106
Solace Association Inc
Tel: 08 272 4334

Tasmania
National Association for Loss
and Grief
144 Albert Road
Moonah 7009
Tel: 002 282 493

Solace Association Inc
Tel: 002 43 8620

Victoria
National Association for Loss
and Grief
PO Box 64
Footscray 3001
Tel: 03 688 4760

Solace Association Inc
Tel: 03 384 1722

Western Australia
National Association for Loss
and Grief
PO Box 110
Fremantle 6160
Tel: 09 443 2697

Solace Association Inc
Tel: 09 332 5863

Nutrition

Australian Capital Territory
Australian Nutrition
Foundation ACT Division
C/-Department of Nutrition
and Dietetics
Royal Canberra Hospital
Acton 2601
Tel: 062 43 2412

New South Wales
Australian Nutrition
Foundation NSW Division
C/- Royal Prince Alfred
Hospital
Missenden Road
Camperdown 2050
Tel: 02 516 6516

Queensland
Australian Nutrition
Foundation Queensland
Division
GPO Box 2734
Brisbane 4001
Tel: 07 229 1503

South Australia
Australian Nutrition
Foundation South Australian.
Division   ·
C/- CSIRO Division of
Human Nutrition
Kintore Avenue
Adelaide 5000
Tel: 08 224 1873

Tasmania
Australian Nutrition
Foundation Tasmania Division
C/-Dr David Woodward
Biochemistry Department,
University of Tasmania
GPO Box 252C
Hobart 7001
Tel: 002 20 2675

Victoria
Australian Nutrition
Foundation Victorian Division
PO Box 185
Caulfield 3162
Tel: 03 528 2453

Western Australia
Australian Nutrition
Foundation WA Division
PO Box 350
Nedlands 6009
Tel: 09 381 6893

Sport and Recreation

National
Minister of Arts, Sport, the
Environment, Tourism and
Territories
GPO Box 787
Canberra 2601

Australian Capital Territory
Life. Be In It
PO Box 1156
Tuggeranong 2900
Tel: 06 293 5630

ACT Office for Sport,
Recreation and Racing
ACT Administration
Centrepoint Building
Anketell Street
Tuggeranong Town Centre
Canberra 2900

New South Wales
Life. Be In It
565 Willoughby Road
Willoughby 2068
Tel: 02 958 6766

Department of Sport and
Recreation
MLC Building
105–53 Miller Street
North Sydney 2060
Tel: 02 923 4234

Department of Health, Senior
Adult Unit
Chattswood District
Community Hospital
PO Box 21
Chattswood 2057

Northern Territory
Life. Be In It
PO Box 1448
Darwin 0801
Tel: 089 82 2325

Office of Youth, Sport,
Recreation and Ethnic Affairs
Sports House
Waratah Crescent
Fannie Bay
Darwin 0800

Queensland
Life. Be In It
PO Box 283
Coorparoo 4151
Tel: 07 394 4444

Division of Sport and
Recreation
Education House
85 George Street
Brisbane 4001

South Australia
Life. Be In It
State Association House
1 Sturt Street
Adelaide 5000
Tel: 08 231 0620

Department of Recreation and
Sport
Citicentre
1 Hindmarsh Square
Adelaide 5000
Tel: 08 234 1724

Tasmania
Life. Be In It
4 Tolosa Street
Glen Orchy 7010
Tel: 002 74 0713

Department of Sport and
Recreation
Kirksway House
Kirksway Place
Battery Point
Hobart 7000
Tel: 002 30 8011

Victoria
Life. Be In It
12 Claremont Street
South Yarra 3141
Tel: 03 826 8222

Department of Sport and
Recreation
123 Lonsdale Street
Melbourne 3000
Tel: 03 666 4200

'Active at Any Age'
Tel: 008 012031

Western Australia
Life. Be In It
PO Box 63
Rivervale 6103
Tel: 09 361 4107

Ministry for Sport and
Recreation
Perry Lakes Stadium
Meagher Drive
Floreat 6001

Education and Learning

Australian Capital Territory
University of the Third Age
Canberra
C/-Hughes Community Centre
Hughes 2605
Tel: 062 82 3777

College of TAFE
Constitution Avenue
Reid 2601
Tel: 062 45 1600

New South Wales
University of the Third Age
Sydney
Centre of Continuing
Education
University of Sydney
Sydney 2006
Tel: 02 692 2567

TAFE Information Centre
849 George Street
Railway Square
Broadway 2007
Tel: 02 212 4400

Australian College for Seniors
The University of Wollongong
PO Box 1144
Wollongong 2500
Tel: 042 270 484

Sydney School for Seniors
13 Wilmont Street
Sydney 2000
Tel: 02 267 8741

Northern Territory
University of the Third Age
PO Box 119

Darwin 0801
Tel: 089 81 7011

Adult Education-TAFE
69 Smith Street
Darwin 0800
Tel: 089 89 5789

Queensland
University of the Third Age
Brisbane
Griffith University
PO Box 82
Mount Gravatt
Tel: 07 875 711

TAFE
1030 Cavendish Road
Mount Gravatt
Tel: 07 343 5988

South Australia
University of the Third Age
Adelaide
28 Franklin Street
Adelaide 5000
Tel: 08 212 6300

Department of TAFE
Information Centre
31 Flinders Street
Adelaide 5000
Tel: 08 226 3409

Tasmania
University of the Third Age
C/- Deputy Vice Chancellor
University of Tasmania
GPO Box 252C
Hobart 7001
Tel: 002 20 2101

Adult Education
452 Elizabeth Street

North Hobart 7000
Tel: 002 30 7326

Victoria
University of the Third Age
Network Victoria
C/- The Council of Adult
Education
256 Flinders Street
Melbourne 3000
Tel: 03 650 1793

TAFE
131 Latrobe Street
Melbourne 3000
Tel: 03 663 5800

Western Australia
University of the Third Age
UWA
University Extension Room
Nedlands 6009
Tel: 09 381 5587

Department of TAFE
Cable House
401 Hay Street
Perth 6000
Tel: 09 325 3544

Independent Living

Australian Capital Territory
Independent Living Centre
Parkinson St
Weston 2611
Tel: 06 287 1644

New South Wales
Independent Living Centre
600 Victoria Road

Ryde 2112
Tel: 02 808 2233

Queensland
Independent Living Centre
Ward 1 Repat. General
Hospital Greenslopes
Newdegate Street
Greenslopes 4120
Tel: 07 394 7471

South Australia
Independent Living Centre
180 Daws Road
Daw Park 5041
Tel: 08 276 3455

Victoria
Independent Living Centre
52 Thistlewaite Street
South Melbourne 3205
Tel: 03 690 9177

Western Australia
Independent Living Centre
3 Lemnos Street
Shenton Park 6008
Tel: 09 382 2011

National Heart Foundation of Australia

National
PO Box 2
Woden ACT 2606
Tel: 062 82 2144

Australian Capital Territory
Royal Insurance Building
25 London Circuit
Canberra ACT 2601
Tel: 062 47 7100

New South Wales
343–9 Riley Street
Surrey Hills 2010
Tel: 02 211 5188

Queensland
557 Gregory Terrace
Fortitude Valley 4006
Tel: 07 854 1696

South Australia
155–9 Hutt Street
Adelaide 5000
Tel: 08 223 3144

Victoria
464 William Street
West Melbourne 3003
Tel: 03 329 8511

Western Australia
43 Stirling Highway
Nedlands 6009
Tel: 09 386 8926

Stroke-Australian Brain Foundation

New South Wales
Burns Philp Building
7 Bridge Street
Sydney 2000
Tel: 02 259 1219

Queensland
Taylor Medical Centre
40 Annerley Road
Woolloongabba 4102
Tel: 07 393 1258

South Australia
31 Franklin Street
Adelaide 5000
Tel: 08 212 5595

Tasmania
'Alkoomi'
St John's Park
New Town 7008
Tel: 002 28 8296

Victoria (and National)
746 Burke Road
Camberwell 3124
Tel: 03 882 2203, 008 33 3469

Western Australia
PO Box 1111
West Perth 6005
Tel: 09 382 2320

Anti-Cancer Councils

Australian Capital Territory
ACT Cancer Society Inc
Health Promotion Centre
15 Theodore Street
Curtin 2605
Tel: 06 285 3070

New South Wales
NSW Cancer Council
Second Floor, Angus and
Coote Building
500 George Street
Sydney 2000
Tel: 02 264 8888

Northern Territory
Norther Territory
Anti-Cancer Foundation
Shop 24, Casuarina Plaza
Casuarina 0810
Tel: 089 27 4888

Queensland
Queensland Cancer Fund

553 Gregory Terrace
Fortitude Valley 4006
Tel: 07 257 1155

South Australia
Anti-Cancer Foundation of
the Universities of South
Australia
24 Brougham Place 5006
Tel: 08 267 5222

Victoria
Anti-Cancer Council of
Victoria
1 Rathdowne Street
Carlton South 3053
Tel: 03 662 3300

Tasmania
Tasmanian Cancer Committee
43 Collins Street
Hobart 7000
Tel: 002 30 0895

Western Australia
Cancer Foundation of WA
(Inc)
42 Ord Street
West Perth 6005
Tel: 09 321 6224, 09 321 2365

Arthritis Foundation

National
Wingella House
Angel Place
Sydney 2000
Tel: 02 221 2456

Australian Capital Territory
Health Promotions Centre
Childers Street
Canberra City 2600

Tel: 06 257 4842

New South Wales
64 Kippax Street
Surrey Hills 2010
Tel: 02 281 1611

Northern Territory
PO Box 37582
Winnellie 0821
Tel: 089 88 1004 (home)

Queensland
Wesley Hospital Grounds
Coronation Drive
Auchenflower 4066
Tel: 07 371 9755

South Australia
99 Anzac Highway
Ashford 5035
Tel: 08 297 2488

Tasmania
30/84 Hampden Road
Battery Point 7000
Tel: 002 34 6489

Victoria
Action House
Yarra Boulevard
Kew 3101
Tel: 03 862 2555

Western Australia
Goatcher House
42 Jersey Street
Jolimont 6014
Tel: 09 387 7066

Diabetes

Australian Capital Territory
Diabetes Australia-ACT

Main Block,
Royal Canberra Hospital
Acton Peninsula
Acton 2601
Tel: 06 247 5211

New South Wales
Diabetes Australia-NSW
149 Pitt Street
Redfern 2016
Tel: 02 698 1100

Northern Territory
Diabetes Australia-NT
2 Tiwi Place
Tiwi 0801
Tel: 089 27 8488

Queensland
Diabetes Australia-Queensland
124 Gerler Road
Hendra 4011
Tel: 07 268 6755

South Australia
Diabetes Australia-SA
157 Burbridge Road
Hilton 5033
Tel: 08 234 1977

Tasmania
Diabetes Australia-Tasmania
65 Davey Street
Hobart 7000
Tel: 002 34 5223

Victoria
Diabetes Australia-Victoria
100 Collins Street
Melbourne 3000
Tel: 03 654 8777

Western Australia
Diabetes Australia-WA

48 Wickham Street
East Perth 6000
Tel: 09 325 7699

Continence Foundation of Australia

Australian Capital Territory
Continence Promotion Group
of the ACT
PO Box 311
Kippax 2615
Tel: 062 54 2555 (Mrs
Chesher)

New South Wales
PO Box 633
Leichhardt 2040
Tel: 02 694 5980 (Dr Millard)

Northern Territory
Casuarina Plaza Health Centre
Casuarina 0810
Tel: 089 20 3211 (Ms Dewar)

Queensland
PO Box 767
Westend 4101
Tel: 07 840 5175 (Mrs
Winnick)

South Australia
C/-SA COTA
23 Coglin Street
Adelaide 5000
Tel: 08 333 0423 (Ms Greene)

Tasmania
Repatriation General Hospital
Hampden Road
Battery Point 7004
Tel: 002 20 9321 (Ms
Sutherland)

Victoria (and National)
First Floor, 449 Swanston
Street
Melbourne 3000
Tel: 03 662 1874

Western Australia
PO Box 591
Claremont 6010
Tel: 09 481 2203 (Mrs
Harrison)

Alzheimer's Disease and Related Disorders Society (ADARDS)

National
ADARDS Australia
PO Box 51
North Ryde 2113
Tel: 02 878 4466

Northern Territory
NT Dementia Worker
AACT
PO Box 40596
Casuarina 0810
Tel: 089 20 3398

Queensland
ADARDA
PO Box 446
Lutwyche 4030
Tel: 07 857 4043

South Australia
ADARDS
PO Box 202
Eastwood 5063
Tel: 08 373 2670

Tasmania
ADARDS
2 St John's Avenue
Newtown 7008
Tel: 002 28 1897

Victoria
ADARDS
84 Eastern Road
South Melbourne 3205
Tel: 03 696 1696

Western Australia
ADARDA WA
C/-Homes of Peace
Subiaco 6008
Tel: 09 388 3800

Parkinson's Disease Associations

National
PO Box 231
Narre Warren, Victoria 3805
Tel: 03 707 1228

Australian Capital Territory
62 Sherbrooke Street
Ainslie 2602
Tel: 062 47 8080

New South Wales
PO Box 2408
North Parramatta 2151
Tel: 02 891 5550

Northern Territory
Darwin Rehab Centre
Tel: 089 81 1877

Queensland
PO Box 521
Lutwyche 4030
Tel: 07 857 1357

South Australia
37 Woodville Road
Woodville 5011
Tel: 08 268 6222

Tasmania
82 Hampten Road
Battery Point 7000
Tel: 002 43 6510

Victoria
583 Ferntree Gully Road
Glen Waverley 3150
Tel: 03 562 0411

Western Australia
5/85 Rokeby Road
Subiaco 6008
Tel: 09 381 8699

Visual Impairment

New South Wales
Royal Blind Society of NSW
PO Box 176
Burwood 2134
Tel: 02 747 6622

Queensland
Royal Blind Society of
Queensland
247 Vulture Street
South Brisbane 4101
Tel: 07 844 4111

South Australia
Royal Society for the Blind of
South Australia
PO Box 196

Greenacres 5086
Tel: 08 261 2611

Victoria
Association for the Blind
7 Mair Street
Brighton Beach 3186
Tel: 03 598 8555

Western Australia
Association for the Blind of
Western Australia
61 Kitchener Avenue
Victoria Park 6100
Tel: 09 362 8202

Hearing Impairment

New South Wales
Better Hearing Australia
288 Unwins Bridge Road
Sydenham 2044
Tel: 02 516 3322

Queensland
Better Hearing Australia
51 Edmondstone Street
South Brisbane 4101
Tel: 07 844 5065

South Australia
Better Hearing Australia
183 Wakefield Street
Adelaide 5000
Tel: 08 232 2996

Tasmania
Better Hearing Australia
29 Second Avenue
West Moonah 7009
Tel: 002 72 0835

Victoria
Better Hearing Australia
5 High Street
Prahran 3181
Tel: 03 510 1577

Western Australia
Better Hearing Australia
29 West Parade
East Perth 6000
Tel: 09 328 7938

FURTHER READING

1. The Ageing Revolution

Kendig, Hal and McCallum, John, *Greying Australia — Future Impacts of Population Ageing*, Australian Government Publishing, Canberra, 1986

Comfort, Alex, *A Good Age*, Pan, London, 1977 (1990 rev. ed.)

Ford, Bruce, *The Elderly Australian*, Penguin, Melbourne, 1979

2. Emotional Challenges

RETIREMENT

Personal Planning and Retirement Kit, Early Planning for Retirement Association, 449 Swanston St., Melbourne 3000, 1990

HOUSING

Banks, Glenda, *Options. A handbook for the elderly and those who care for them*, Dove Communications, Melbourne, 1984

Wilson, Pam and Calder, Rosemary, *Housing choices for older Australians*, Australian Council on the Ageing, Melbourne, 1990

Zeigler Harriet, *It's Your Move*, Wesley Central Mission, Melbourne, 1985

SEXUALITY

Masters, William, Johnson, Virginia and Kolody, Robert, *Masters and Johnson on Sex and Human Loving*, Macmillan, London, 1982

Butler, Robert and Lewis, Myrna, *Love and Sex after 60*, Harper and Rowe, New York, 1976

CARING
Schultz, Noel and Cynthia, *The Key to Caring*, Longman Cheshire, Melbourne, 1990

DEATH
McKissock, Mal, *Coping with grief*, Australian Broadcasting Commission, Sydney, 1987
Kubler-Ross, Elizabeth, *On Death & Dying*, Macmillan, New York, 1969

3. Exercise

Gibbs, Russell, *Exercise for the over–50s*, Sun Books, Melbourne, 1981
Wicks, John, *Guide to Exercise*, National Heart Foundation of Australia, Melbourne

4. Food and Nutrition

Gaté, Gabriel, *Smart Food*, Anne O'Donovan, Melbourne, 1989
Gaté, Gabriel, *Good Food Fast. High energy low fuss family food*, Anne O'Donovan, Melbourne, 1991
Morgan, Wendy and Pomeroy, Sylvia, *Cooking For Few—A quide for easy cooking for one or two*, National Heart Foundation, Melbourne, 1988
Saxelby, Catherine, *Nutrition for Life*, Reed Books, Sydney, 1986

5. Stress and Relaxation

Montgomery, Bob and Evans, Lynette, *You & Stress, A guide to Successful Living*, Viking O'Neil, Melbourne, 1984
Davis, Martha, Eshelman, Elizabeth and McKay, Mathew, *The Relaxation and Stress Reduction Workbook*, New Harbinger Publications, Oakland, 1983
Downing, George, *The Massage Book*, Penguin, London, 1986
Ellis, Albert and Harper, Robert, *A New Guide to Rational Living*, Wilshire Book Company, North Hollywood/California, 1975

Mears, Ainsley, *Relief Without Drugs*, Fontana/Collins, Glasgow, 1968

Mears, Ainsley, *Why be Old? How to avoid the psychological reactions of Ageing*, Hill of Content, Melbourne, 1980

7. Prevention

Hetzel, Basil and McMichael, Tony, *The LS Factor*, Penguin, Melbourne, 1987

Rosenfeld, Isadore, *Modern Prevention, The New Medicine*, Bantam Books, New York, 1987

HEART

Borushek, Alan, *The Complete Australian Heart Disease Prevention Manual*, Family Health Publication, West Perth, 1981

OBESITY

Tupling, Hilary, *A Weight Off Your Mind*, Bantam Books, Sydney, 1991

MENOPAUSE

Llewllyn-Jones, Derek and Abrahams, Suzanne, *Menopause*, Penguin, Melbourne, 1988

OSTEOPOROSIS

Cooper, Wendy, *Understanding Osteoporosis*, Arrow Books, London, 1990

INCONTINENCE

Millard, Richard, *Bladder Control, a Simple Self-Help Guide*, Williams & Wilkens and Associates, Sydney, 1987

Fonda, David and Wellings, Cynthia, *Urinary Incontinence. A practical guide for people with bladder problems, their carers and health care professionals*, AGCD Publishing, Melbourne, 1987

DEMENTIA

Mace, Nancy and Rabins, Peter, *The 36 Hour Day: A Family Guide to Caring for Persons with Alzheimer's Disease and Related Dementing Illnesses*, John Hopkins University Press, Baltimore, 1981

Naughton, Gerry and Laidler, Terry, *When I Grow Too Old to Dream. Coping with Alzheimer's Disease*, Collins Dove, Melbourne, 1991

SLEEPLESSNESS
Wong, Moses, *Sleep Without Drugs*, Hill of Content, Melbourne, 1989

INDEX